The New Lean Healthcare Pocket Guide XL

Tools for the Elimination of Waste in Hospitals, Clinics, and Other Healthcare Facilities

D0290099

© 2010 by MCS Media, Inc.

All rights reserved. No part of this book may be reproduced or utilized in any form or by any means, electronic or mechanical, including photocopying, recording, or by any information storage and retrieval system, without permission in writing from the publisher.

ISBN 978-0-9825004-5-3

07 06 05 04 03   5 4 3 2 1

Contents

🍎 Denotes Case Studies and/or Photos

Acknowledgements

Our sincere thanks goes out to the people who reviewed previous versions of this pocket guide as well as contributing to this newer version.

Rita D'Angelo is currently the quality improvement specialist in the Department of Pathology and Laboratory Medicine in the Henry Ford Health System, Detroit Michigan, where she is in charge of process redesign in the 12th largest hospital-based laboratory in the country.

Richard Zarbo, MD is the chair and senior vice-president of Pathology and Laboratory Medicine in the Henry Ford Health System. He is a board certified anatomic and clinical pathologist and an expert in head and neck pathology, who has been instrumental in defining benchmarks of laboratory quality over the past 18 years. Dr. Zarbo is the president of the United States and Canadian Academy of Pathology.

Ruan Varney, CT, ASQ CQE, SSBB is the Quality Improvement Coordinator in the Department of Pathology and Laboratory Medicine for Henry Ford Health System. She is a graduate of Diagnostic Cytopathology from Toronto Canada. In the past she has coordinated a study of Improving Patient Safety by Examining Pathology Errors for AHRQ (Agency for Healthcare Research and Quality). She holds certificates in Quality Engineer and Six Sigma Black Belt from American Society for Quality.

Cindy Allen-Fedor, RN

Michael Blatchford, Lean Sensei

Marty Holmes, MD

Gale Easton, PA - C

Rob Ptacek, Lean Sensei

Publisher's Message

As Yogi Berra once said, "The future isn't what it used to be." Currently, healthcare facilities are challenged to improve the quality of care, improve staff/patient satisfaction, as well as balance the budget. Insurance and governmental programs have cut back on allocations to the healthcare community. Increased technology costs and the number of people with no healthcare coverage make the struggle more challenging than ever. Meanwhile, people are more concerned than ever about escalating healthcare costs given the economic meltdown and the unemployment rate that has impacted nearly every man, woman, and child. The net effect is that healthcare facilities must find innovative and simple ways to improve patient care and safety while controlling costs. Hospitals, clinics, and labs across the United States and Canada, and throughout the world, have found success in using the Toyota Production System (i.e., Lean) as a business improvement tool in meeting those challenges.

The Lean tools are all here, functionally described and illustrated for ease of adaptation and usage to:

- Identify and eliminate waste quickly and efficiently in any hospital, lab, or clinic
- Increase participation and communication at all levels of the facility
- Create standardize processes
- Create a favorable environment allowing a continuous improvement culture to emerge

The New Lean Healthcare Pocket Guide XL was developed for all staff levels within a healthcare organization. This insightful and ready-to-use guide can be your path to improved patient safety, increased efficiency, and reduced stress!

Don Tapping

About the Authors

Debra K. Hadfield, RN, MSN, CFPN has worked in the clinical, hospital, and educational fields applying Lean Healthcare principles for over ten years. Ms. Hadfield has held positions at Michigan State University, The University of Michigan, Andrews University, Michigan Capital Medical Center, and Battle Creek Family Practice.

Shelagh Holmes, RN, has 22 years of nursing experience. Ms. Holmes has held a wide range of healthcare positions, including: emergency room nurse, nurse manager, consolidation program manager, university instructor, labor coach, and medical clinic manager.

Todd Sperl is a Master Black Belt/Lean Sensei and led the deployment of Lean-Six Sigma across St. John Health. His experience ranges from facilitating large, complex organizational transformation initiatives to achieve significant and measurable results, as well as participating on numerous smaller engagements. Currently Todd is Managing Partner at Lean Fox Solutions, LLC, a healthcare consulting firm where their vision is to improve the patient care experience. Todd can be contacted at tsperl@leanfoxsolutions.com.

Susan F. Kozlowski, MSA, MT(ASCP) SBB DLM, CSSBB (ASQ) was one of the first Lean Six Sigma Black Belts at St. John Health completing numerous projects in areas of inpatient flow, bed management, the Emergency Department, Surgical Services, and Registration. Sue is currently the Manager of Performance Improvement at Henry Ford Hospital in Detroit. Certified as a Black Belt by ASQ, Sue is an active member and has served as a judge for the International Team Excellence Awards.

Visit **www.theleanstore.com** for workshop information on conducting a Lean healthcare workshop at your facility.

How to Use *The New Lean Healthcare Pocket Guide XL*

The New Lean Healthcare Pocket Guide XL is designed for use as a convenient and quick reference as you learn and implement the Lean tools as they apply to those challenging situations in healthcare. You can put your finger on any tool within a matter of seconds!

Find the right tool for the right Lean initiative by using either the Table of Contents, the Lean Healthcare Tool Usage Matrix or the Index.

- **Table of Contents** offers an alphabetical list of tools, techniques, and supporting information.

- **Lean Healthcare Tool Usage Matrix** organizes the Lean tools and concepts relative to important broad Lean philosophies.

The philosophies are:

Stabilize - It is critical that excess movement of work and variation of process be removed first. It is difficult to apply Lean when variation exists.

Standardize - Once an area or a process has been stabilized, formal standards via work rules, charts, and visual controls must be used to further eliminate variation.

Simplify - As an organization stabilizes and standardizes processes, it must work to level the work loads among staff to ensure effective and efficient service is provided to the patient or other healthcare provider.

- **Index** will provide a quick access to a specific topic or tool.

As you continue with the implementation of Lean initiatives throughout this pocket guide, *assess, diagnosis, treat,* and *prevent* will be the overriding themes.

What do the icons signify?

The Lean journey is similar to the treatment of a patient. It requires people (healthcare providers and staff) and support from various departments and ancillary staff to effectively apply Lean concepts and tools. As the treatment of a patient is individually tailored, Lean must also be tailored to the facility, department, and/or process in which it will be used. Throughout this guide, specific icons will alert you to the four themes of: *Assess, Diagnosis, Treat,* and *Prevent.* These icons are represented as follows:

Assess - This is the most critical step in Lean healthcare. In medicine, professional skills are used to assess and evaluate a patient. In Lean, similar assessment skills are used to evaluate an area or process and prepare it for detailed analysis. This involves teamwork represented by the icon of team members reviewing a productivity measurement. Each member of the team plays a vital role, bringing to the table different skills. In this section, expect a brief description of the tool's purpose, who is mainly responsible for doing it, and how long it will take to implement.

Diagnosis - Just as a stethoscope assists in determining a diagnosis of a patient, Lean tools are used to identify and gather information for adequate measurements to be taken. This also involves teamwork, as a diagnosis is often reached using a multi-disciplinary approach. This allows a statement or conclusion to be drawn concerning the nature or cause of the area or process requiring attention. In this section, expect a brief description of what this tool will do. This will provide the transition from assessing an area or process through further analysis and understanding to ensuring the correct treatment (or action) is taken.

Treat - The prescription pad represents treatment after the assessment and diagnosis have been completed.

In the Lean process, treatment involves the application of a Lean tool to a process or area. In medicine, the ultimate goal is to achieve wellness for a patient. In Lean, the goal is to attain a state of continuous improvement. In this section, you will find detailed steps that are to be implemented for the use of this tool. It will also provide key points.

Prevent - "An apple a day keeps the doctor away." This implies preventing illness and sustaining health.

In healthcare, prevention is the key to the ultimate goal of wellness. Lean tools are applied to ensure Total Employee Involvement (TEI) and to sustain the gains that were achieved. In this section (of most chapters) you will find case studies and actual photos conveying successful applications of that particular Lean tool or practice. This sharing will allow you to prevent waste in similar-type activities related to your Lean or Six Sigma project.

These icons will be your navigator and will provide guidance in your Lean or Six Sigma journey. Even though the concepts are referred to as Lean, they will support any type of improvement project (i.e., Six Sigma, TQM, etc.).

Most importantly, keep in mind that many Lean tools compliment each other. Rarely will only one tool be used by itself.

Waste in Healthcare

Any time a process exists, there is the potential for waste or non value-added activities. Healthcare, like all other industries, is comprised of many processes.

HealthMEDX, a provider of information system solutions for the extended care market, reports the following:

"For every dollar spent on healthcare, over 75 cents is spent on the non-patient care activities of communicating, scheduling, coordinating, supervising, and documenting care."

In an article in Industry Week, published November 1, 2003, a nurse medical researcher stated:

"The national numbers for waste in healthcare are between 30% and 40%, but the reality of what we've observed doing minute-by-minute observation over the last three years is closer to 60%. That's a waste of time, waste of money, waste of material resources. The waste is not limited to administrative costs, which most research on healthcare spending has documented. It's everywhere: patient care and non-patient care alike."

Lean eliminates waste or non value-added activities. Waste is defined through the eyes of the customer and includes anything that does not add value to the final product or service, and all activities that customers are not willing to pay for. For example, a patient does not want to pay for a second surgical tray if only one instrument was used from it.

Non value-added activities are usually symptoms of a problem within a process. Non value-added activities increase costs by using time and resources without directly satisfying the needs of the customer. Value-added activities, on the other hand, are those things customers (i.e., typically the patient) are willing to pay for, including a medication that makes them feel better or the results of an MRI that enable his or her physician to provide treatment. Value-added activities satisfy customers by directly fulfilling their needs.

There are eight categories of waste in healthcare:

1. Unnecessary services or overproduction
2. Mistakes or defects
3. Delays or waiting
4. Unnecessary motion or movement
5. Overprocessing
6. Excess inventory
7. Excess transport
8. Unused creativity

You will find a closer examination of these eight categories contained in the Waste section of this book. Each waste is explained in detail. Examples are provided on how these wastes are manifested within healthcare processes. Once the concept of waste is understood, it becomes easier to diagnose its presence, apply treatment, and improve its condition through the use of Lean practices and principles.

A Lean Perspective

Lean, the Toyota Production System, waste elimination, and process/continuous improvement are used synonymously. Lean is a compilation of world-class practices that will improve an organization through an evidence-based methodology.

The purpose of Lean is to eliminate all waste or non value-added activities from a process. The focus on the elimination of waste should be a daily, hourly, or minute-by-minute review. Lean is not meant to eliminate people, but to use them more wisely. With that thought in mind, job duties (tasks) may need to be modified to accommodate a waste-free (Lean) environment. This will allow healthcare facilities to improve patient safety and care while creating a culture of continuous improvement.

Lean is based on reducing costs rather than raising prices (or reducing services).

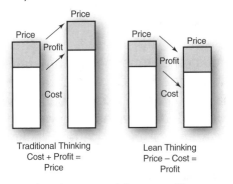

Traditional Thinking
Cost + Profit =
Price

Lean Thinking
Price – Cost =
Profit

A healthcare organization must be run like a successful business, focusing on achieving a positive Return-On-Investment (ROI) by eliminating, or at least minimizing, non value-added activities through the implementation of Lean practices. These practices will deliver new, non-traditional approaches to reducing waste and improving healthcare. This is accomplished through this proactive cost and process improvement methodology.

Why Lean in Healthcare

The current healthcare system must improve due to the enormous defect rate (estimated at nearly 45% by the New England Journal of Medicine, June 26, 2003), premium cost escalation, nursing shortages, etc. General Motors Corporation reported that healthcare expenditures equate to $1,525 per car. This costs more than the steel to make the car! The insult to injury is that a significant portion of the costs related to healthcare services is waste. The national numbers for waste in healthcare are between 30 and 40%.

The good news is that significant innovations are available to eliminate this waste and improve institutional function. This is achieved through the adaptation of the world-class processes that have been documented and used by the Toyota Motor Corporation (i.e., Lean).

Lean is centered around eliminating waste through continuous improvement while always keeping the customer in mind. Waste is defined as non value-added activities that the customer is unwilling to pay for. Non value-added activities are the inefficiencies within the process. The service or product provided to the customer must be what the customer is willing to pay for (value-added). Doctor appointments, where a patient might have an X-ray taken, blood drawn, etc., are an example of value-added activities. However, the functions of patient charting, transporting a patient, billing, coding, etc., may appear as non value-added, but are necessary to ensure total patient satisfaction and safety. Therefore, as we discuss eliminating waste (or non value-activities), be careful to not refer to these as non value-added activities. They are essential services required for patient safety and care.

The ultimate customer is the patient, but remember, internal customers can be physicians, other staff, departments, vendors, or healthcare providers.

Ultimate Case Studies for Lean in Healthcare

ED-Orthopedics

The Oak Valley Medical Center experienced delays and significant patient dissatisfaction in their Emergency Room, specifically their orthopedic patient services. This was determined by their annual patient survey. The Chief of Staff and Nurse Coordinator from the ER department attended a Lean healthcare workshop to explore ways to improve their services. Subsequently, they decided that the Lean process could improve this particular part of the facility. The day after the workshop, an improvement team was formed consisting of staff from various departments and disciplines. The team created a Team Charter and decided to collect additional data on the Orthopedic Patient Visit value stream. (See Reporting and Communications, Document Tagging, and Cycle Time)

After collecting the additional data and implementing problem solving, a current state value stream map was created. Reviewing the past 3 months of records, it was determined that an average of 6 orthopedic patients were seen in the ER room for casting during a 12 hour shift. This created a takt time of 2 hours for this value stream. The measurements of cycle times, wait times, and lead times were established for this value stream. (See Takt Time, Waste, Value Stream Mapping, and Problem Solving)

See the next page for the Orthopedic Patient Current State Value Stream Map for the Emergency Room.

Orthopedic Patient Current State Value Stream Map for the Emergency Room

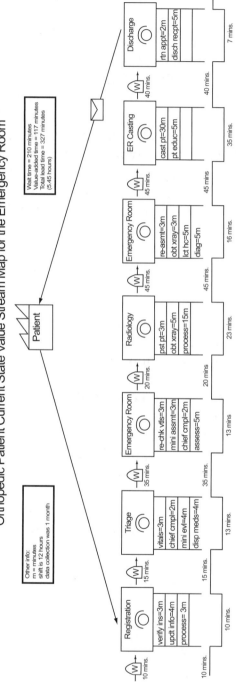

Other info:
m = minutes
shift is 12 hours
data collection was 1 month

Wait time = 210 minutes
Value-added time = 117 minutes
Total lead time = 327 minutes
(5.45 hours)

Registration
verify ins=3m
updt info=4m
process= 3m

Triage
vitals=3m
chief cmpl=2m
mini evl=4m
disp meds=4m

Emergency Room
re-chk vtls=3m
mini assmt=3m
chief cmpl=2m
assess=5m

Radiology
pst pt=3m
obt xray=5m
process=15m

Emergency Room
re-asmt=3m
obt xray=3m
lct hc=5m
diag=5m

ER Casting
cast pt=30m
pt educ=5m

Discharge
rtn appt=2m
disch recpt=5m

10 mins. — 15 mins. — 35 mins. — 20 mins. — 45 mins. — 45 mins. — 40 mins.

10 mins. — 15 mins. — 13 mins — 20 mins. — 23 mins. — 45 mins. — 16 mins. — 45 mins. — 35 mins. — 40 mins. — 7 mins.

13 mins

The team brainstormed and determined the following kaizen events: (See Kaizen Event)

1. Work load balancing and cross-training would be used between the Triage nurse and the Emergency Room (ER) nurse. In the current state, the Triage nurse performed vitals, recorded Chief Complaint (CC), performed brief initial evaluation, and dispensed pain medications. In the future state, they decided to eliminate the wait time between Triage and the first ER encounter. This was accomplished by taking the patient directly from the Triage to the ER suite due to the obvious need for treatment. The vitals, assessment, etc. would not be repeated at this time. This eliminated many steps of the initial ER room visit. Both the Triage nurse and ER nurse would be cross-trained and qualified. This had required the Triage nurse to be trained in ER nursing. Also, the initial wait time at registration was to be eliminated by creating a placard for the patient to begin filling in initial information. (See Work Load Balancing and Standard Work)

2. Kanban for supplies would be used in the ER medication room. This would create a Pull System for the supplies. The current state had the nurse searching for a 3 cc syringe, along with the ordered medications. This caused a delay in patient care delivery. The future state would implement kanbans, which ensured the supplies were well stocked and available when needed. (See Pull System and Kanbans for Supplies)

3. Visual controls would be used to notify the nurse of patient room availability and the location of the healthcare provider. In the current state, the ER nurse searched for the healthcare provider while also looking for an available room, which caused additional delay. The future state eliminated this searching for the healthcare provider and room by installing a multi-color light system. This eliminated the queue time between Triage and the initial ER encounter. (See Visual Controls)

4. Each ER suite had supplies missing from various areas. This caused the nurse to become frustrated and led to time delays in caring for patients from one suite to another. The future state incorporated the 5S process to eliminate this problem. (See 5S)

5. The current state had a delay of 30 minutes from the second ER encounter to the Casting Room. In the future state, the Triage nurse will be notifying the Casting Room technician via a visual control (i.e., pager code number) that a patient will be requiring his or her services within a 30 minute period. Previously the Casting Room technician would be notified at the time the cast was to be applied, which resulted in a wait time of 30 minutes. The Casting Room staff used 5S to better organize their room. Because of the early notifications and better room (bed) assignments, they were now more prepared to receive a patient within 15 minutes. (See Visual Controls)

6. The current state had the physical layout utilizing the Radiology department for the majority of cases requiring X-rays. This had caused a delay of 20 minutes. In the future state, a portable radiology unit and technician (runner) were utilized in the ER suite. This eliminated the transport to and from Radiology and the respective wait times. (See Physical Layout and Runner)

7. Once the future state was fully implemented, everyone was trained in the new processes. This resulted in a change for many staff. Subsequently, a "lunch and learn" was conducted to educate the staff on the changes being made. (See Resistance to Change)

The team created a future state value stream map to visually convey these changes.

See the next page for the Orthopedic Patient Future State Value Stream Map for the Emergency Room.

Orthopedic Patient Future State Value Stream Map for the Emergency Room

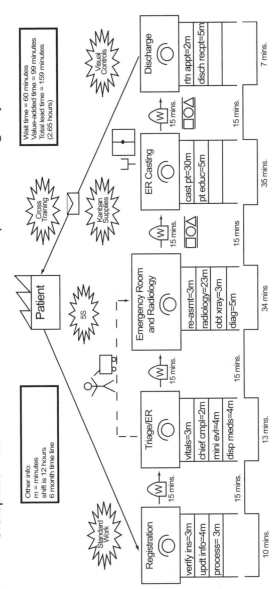

The team implemented the future state in six months. A mini-survey was conducted and the ER Orthopedic services far exceeded any departmental scores. Also, supply costs were reduced by 22%, patient throughput increased by 12%, and nurse satisfaction increased as well. Throughout the implementation the team was looking forward to a new future state that included the following strategies: Leveling, Paper (Chart) File System, Just-In-Time, Takt Time, Pitch, and Predictable Output.

EMR in a Physician's Group

As more healthcare organizations implement an Electronic Medical Record system (or EMR as it is sometimes called), there is a need to design efficient processes that support the most effective use of these computer-based applications. Lean is a perfect partner to this type of process change. As the old saying goes, we do not want to "automate a bad process." The process itself must be analyzed, reviewed, and improved upon to take full advantage of the benefit that an EMR system can provide.

A high volume, Orthopedic Surgeon practice in the Midwest implemented an EMR solution designed for orthopedic workflows. This solution was designed to better utilize resources, improve communication between medical staff, and provide physicians with fast access to patient medical records and images. While the group experienced notable cost savings around the reduction of paperwork and efficiency accessing medical records, they did not witness improved efficiency related to patient throughput.

A cross section of the office staff was engaged to develop a current state process map, including the office manager, front desk associates, X-ray technicians, medical assistants, practice director, and one of the group's surgeons to determine not only why patient throughput had not improved, but what can be done to improve it. The current state map indicated to the group that the patient/work flow did not change after implementation of the EMR system.

The team, realized that eliminating process waste, creating continuous flow, building quality at the source, stabilizing and standardizing processes, using visual controls, and engaging and respecting everyone's contribution were needed to improve efficiencies related to patient throughput.

The time between the patient's initial contact with the office to their appointment varied greatly (e.g., 24 hours to one week) which was mainly due to the patient's and/or physician's availability and the patient experience from the time they entered the office until the time they left. Data over a 3 day period, captured from the EMR system showed the average office visit was 60 minutes with a standard deviation of 19 minutes. For the purpose of this case study, the team focused on the patient's experience for one orthopedic surgeon.

After mapping out the process and capturing some initial data, the team continued with their Lean analysis of the office and the patient's experience. Additional questions that were asked of the staff about the information flow were:

- Does everyone know the hourly patient target?
- How quickly are problems and abnormalities in the schedule noticed?
- What happens when there are problems and abnormalities?
- Does the patient move smoothly from one value-added step to the next?

To assist in answering the last question - Does the patient move smoothly from one value-added step to the next? - the team created a Spaghetti Map to show the flow of the patient. The triangles represent where delays were occurring in the patient's experience as shown below.

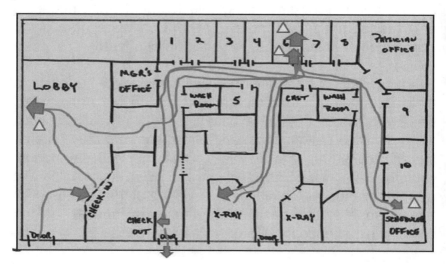

The team was amazed on how much the patient traveled through this process. They also commented that if Spaghetti Maps were completed for the medical assistant, X-ray technician, and physician, then similar type travel would be indicated. Further discussions with the team members revealed the following:

- There were variations in each major step of the patient experience, including the operations of check-in, X-ray, exam, and discharge.
- Operations were isolated (or decoupled) allowing the batching of patients instead of one piece flow from each other. This inherently created the waste of waiting into each step along the way.
- Decoupled operations also made it difficult to notice problems as they happen. None of the work areas (i.e., stations) were aware of problems as they occurred, therefore, everyone kept working. By the end of the day, the unnoticed problems added up and the subsequent length of the patient stay continually fell short of the target.

THE NEW LEAN HEALTHCARE POCKET GUIDE XL

Based on the initial assessment of the process, as well as further diagnosis, the team implemented the following Lean tools:

Introduced a Pull System. Nothing is done by the upstream process until the downstream customer signals the need, e.g., the patient is "pulled" into the X-ray process once an exam room is opened. The EMR becomes the trigger (i.e., kanban or signal). A computer screen visually shows when the "room" in the EMR turns gray which alerts the X-ray technician to "pull" the next patient back.

Standard Work. The completed paperwork for each patient varied greatly depending on which representative scheduled the appointment or how prepared the patient was to answer basic insurance and/or medical history questions. Additionally, while most patients have access to the internet and could complete critical paperwork prior to their visit, they were not always directed to the group's website to download necessary forms, e.g., new patient, insurance, etc. To add to this most patients were arriving close to their scheduled appointment time, but then would have to spend an additional 20 to 30 minutes completing paperwork. (Note this time is additional to the EMR captured data). This pattern caused the office to run behind from the start without the ability to catch up. The standard work solutions included a scripted process for gathering critical data:

1. Encourage patient to access and complete critical medical history and insurance forms on the physician group's website. Noting that if not completed before their appointment their office visit would be longer than anticipated.

2. If the patient did not have access to the internet and there was enough lead time the forms would be mailed directly to the patient for them to complete before their visit. If the patient did not have access to the internet and there was not enough lead time to mail necessary forms to their house the Call Center representatives would try to capture the data immediately or schedule time for them to reconnect with the patient.

3. The final option would be for the patient to arrive 20 to 30 minutes before scheduled appointment to complete necessary paperwork. Depending on the physician and/or the X-ray technician's experience different types of X-rays were being ordered for similar procedures. For example, a simple knee injury might see 3 to 6 different X-rays ordered depending on the physician and or X-ray technician (overproduction). To minimize this confusion and eliminate potential rework, specific procedures by product line were developed to eliminate any discrepancies surrounding specific X-ray requests, e.g., new hip patient requires AP/Lateral Lumbar Spine, AP Pelvis and AP/Lateral.

Continuous Patient Flow and Physical Layout. To minimize the number of steps and improve patient flow two major changes were made to the office. First, the team decided to move the Scheduler's office to the front and place the Manager in the Scheduler's old office. Second, the team changed the flow of the patient which allowed the patient to be X-rayed before going to the exam room. These two changes minimized the congestion in the hallways thus reducing the number of steps a patient was required to complete during their visit.

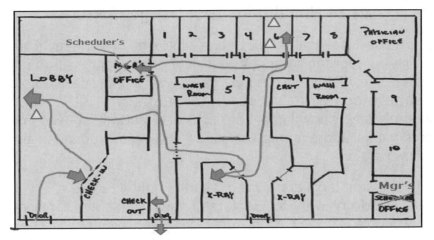

The improvements dramatically decrease the amount of time a patient spends in the office, thus improving patient throughput. Before and after results are shown below:

Patient Experience	Visits	Average	Std Dev
Pre-Pilot	136	1:00	:19
Pilot	133	:29	:14

Moving forward the team focused on deploying the future state across all physician clinics, i.e., the Spinal and Ortho areas and the Call Center.

Note: The Lean tools presented in these two case studies represented one course of action given the particulars of each of the cases.

Lean Healthcare Tool Usage Matrix

The Lean Healthcare Tool Usage Matrix guides a healthcare facility in applying the right Lean tool or concept at the right time. The matrix on the next page was created to promote understanding that these Lean tools are very much interrelated. Many times more than one tool will be used in a continuous improvement activity. The matrix provides the following:

1. Ensures tools are utilized with the right intent (e.g., you would not want to create standard work without having people involved in the data collection of process cycle times)

2. Raises awareness that many tools require teamwork from staff (Total Employee Involvement)

3. Creates an understanding of the three-phase approach of Stabilize, Standardize, and Simplify for implementation

4. Identifies which sections have case studies and/or actual photos

Use the matrix as a guide, checklist, or template for brainstorming. It will help you apply the right tool, at the right time, and in the right way!

Lean Healthcare Tool Usage Matrix

Lean Tool	Levels for Use			Guidelines					Examples
	Stabilize	Standardize	Simplify	General	Assess	Diagnosis	Treat	Prevent	Case Studies and/or Photos
5S in Healthcare - Why You Need It	X				X				Page 13
Continuous Flow	X						X		Page 24
Cycle Time	X					X			Page 30
Document Tagging	X					X			
Error Proofing			X					X	Page 42
Goals and Outcomes	X	X	X		X			X	
Goal Card	X	X	X	X					Page 56
Healthcare Case for Lean				X					Page 63
Interruptions and Random Arrivals					X				
Just-In-Time	X			X					
Kaizen Events	X	X	X	X			X		Page 75
Kanbans for Supplies							X		Page 83
Leveling			X				X		Page 89
Measurement Techniques	X				X				
Paper File System		X					X		Page 108
Physical Layout		X					X		
Pitch			X				X		Page 117
Predictable Output	X			X					
Problem Solving	X	X	X	X	X	X	X	X	Page 137
Pull Systems		X		X					Page 144
Reporting and Communications	X	X	X	X					
Resistance to Change	X			X					
Runners		X					X		
Six Sigma	X	X	X	X	X	X	X	X	Page 166
Standard Work		X					X	X	Page 171
Takt Time	X				X				
Value Stream Mapping				X	X				Page 185
Visual Controls	X	X	X	X	X	X	X	X	Page 194
Waste	X	X	X	X	X	X	X	X	
Work Load Balancing		X					X		Page 211

5S in Healthcare - Why You Need It

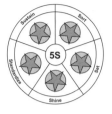

Why use it?

5S is a process to ensure work areas are systematically kept clean and organized, which assures staff and patient safety. It also provides the foundation on which to build a Lean healthcare environment. 5S is an improvement process to ensure everything has a place and everything is in its place. This leads to improved patient and information flow, decreased cost for the facility, and the elimination of time spent searching for things, which is a waste.

The five steps in the process are:

1st S - for **sorting** the necessary from the unnecessary.
When in doubt, move it out!
2nd S - for planning the best place to **set** items in order.
To ensure everything has a place and everything is in its place!
3rd S - for **shining**, cleaning, and identifying items.
To be Lean, you must be clean!
4th S - for creating and setting the **standards** for cleanliness.
Standardize to improve!
5th S - for establishing the discipline to **sustain** the first 4 S's through education and communication.
Sustain the gains!

Who does it?

A temporary Lean team is normally established to initiate and monitor 5S implementation. All employees will be responsible for contributing to the 5S process.

How long will it take?

Depending on the healthcare area, each "S" could take only a few hours to begin with, then a couple minutes per day/per staff member to maintain.

 ## What does it do?

It provides a structured approach and easy-to-understand methodology (steps) for departmental organization, order, and cleanliness. This is accomplished by:

- Placing a team of healthcare professionals in control of their own workplace
- Helping a team and facility focus on the causes of waste and its subsequent elimination
- Establishing standards for basic organization and orderliness
- Demonstrating to patients and staff (co-workers) that a clean environment is a foundation for good work flow
- Improving staff morale by ensuring the area is safe, clean, and something to be proud of

How do you do it?

A cross-functional team is assembled and a target area is chosen. Staff from the work area are key in making this project a success. It is essential to obtain upper management involvement. Mention benefits such as: potential savings of staff's time and other facility efficiencies.

1st S Sort through and sort out.
When in doubt, move it out!

This is the weeding out of items in the target area (a specific physical area of the facility) that have not been used for a period of time and/or are not expected to be used. The team and/or staff member would follow these steps:

a. Define the staging area (physical area to place items that will need to be further categorized).

b. Create the Sort Inspection Sheet for items not essential to the area(s). (It is recommended that if an item has not been touched in 3 months it should be removed from the area.)

Sort Inspection Sheet

Purpose: To ensure that everyone examines all potential items for Sort.

Who Should Fill It Out: A selected team member as areas are reviewed for Sort.

Directions: The best way to use this tool is to follow these steps:
1. Examine all areas under each category for the entire target area.
2. Remove the unneeded item from the area and attach a tag.

Search these spaces:
Floors
Aisles
Desktops
Stairs
Corners/behind desks, beds, and equipment
Interior drawers, cabinets, under counters
Closets
Supply rooms
Locker rooms
Chart carts

Look for unneeded or excess furniture:
Chairs
Gurneys
Beds
Carts
Filing cabinets
Wheelchairs
Side tables in lobby
Bedside trays
Refrigerators
Unused display cases
Unused med cabinets
Damaged equipment

Look for unneeded or excess equipment:
Computers
Printers
Phones
Copiers
IV poles
Crutches and canes
Office supplies

Check the walls, boards, etc:
Outdated hanging and posted items
Old calendars
Useless signboards
Unused message boards
Outdated CME memos

Look for excess supplies:
Medicine Cups
Syringes
Needles
Gloves
Paper and old charts
Pens, scissors, tape, etc.
Outdated or duplicated manuals, pamphlets, and/or drug books
Old lab coats or scrubs
Outdated or unused models (skeletons)

Search these storage areas:
Bookshelves for outdated books
Closets
Drug storage areas
Cupboards and cabinets
Refrigerators
Supply cabinet carts

Look for other unneeded items:
Mugs and old dishes
Trash cans
Broken, unused, or excess equipment
Vacuums, brooms, and/or mops
Condiments in drawers

---

c. Identify items that are not necessary in the area and tag them.

Name:

Date:

Location of Item:

Reason for Tagging:

d. Locate items to a staging area. A staging area is a physical location that items are placed after having been tagged.

e. Managers/Team Leaders determine disposition of tagged items. This may include: return to area, dispose of, or donate to a school or charity.

f. Post the 5S visual circle in a common area and place a seal on the first S.

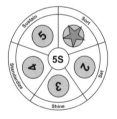

2nd S **Set** things in order and set limits.

To ensure everything has a place and everything is in its place!

This S establishes the locations where items belong, by either labeling or visual markings. The team and/or staff member would follow these steps:

a. Mark off common areas, label drawers, and identify everything within the area.

b. Create a Criteria Checklist for Set-In-Order to assist the team in arranging items.

	Criteria Checklist for Set-In-Order
Team Members: _____	
Purpose: To assist in brainstorming as the future state is created.	
Target Area: _____ **Date:** _____	

	Consider These Questions
1	Can multiple items be grouped and placed in the same location?
2	Can work be arranged so backups do not occur?
3	Can work, service, and/or information exchanges occur in a straight line?
4	Have desktops and common areas been considered?
5	Is all the furniture required for the target area?
6	Is all the equipment being used regularly in the target area?
7	Are the "more often" used items stored near point-of-use?
8	Can items that do not need to be in the immediate area have a visual control?
9	Can heavier items be stored at waist level for ergonomic reasons?
10	Can the First-In First-Out rule apply to supplies and equipment?
11	Do cupboards need doors?
12	Can everything be labeled so anyone can locate it within 5 seconds?
13	Do the equipment and supplies have a practical and current purpose?
14	Does the layout allow for information and equipment to be easily accessible?
15	
16	
17	
18	
19	

c. Create a standard for the target area, something to refer to if an item is out of place or not returned. It should be obvious if something is missing. Each item should be labeled to identify where it belongs.

d. Monitor the area to ensure this S is being completed.

e. Post the 5S visual circle in a common area and place a seal on the second S.

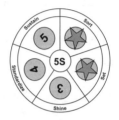

3rd S **Shine** and inspect through cleaning.
   To be Lean, you must be clean!

This is basic cleaning of the area and establishing the sequence in which the area should be maintained on a regular basis. This ranges from cleaning the phone receiver to disposing of expired medications. The team should do a "spring cleaning" and then create a Cleaning Plan. The team and/or staff member would follow these steps:

   a. Conduct a "spring-cleaning" activity.
   b. Create the 5S Cleaning Plan for the area, which may be done daily, weekly, etc.

5S Cleaning Plan				
Department _____			**Date** _____	
Location	5S Task	Name	Frequency	Materials

   c. Post the 5S visual circle in a common area and place a seal on the third S.

5S is a team process but it also requires the individual staff member to commit to the process for his/her own area. It is critical to identify what needs to be cleaned, how often it should be cleaned, and by whom, while using a visual aid (i.e., form or chart).

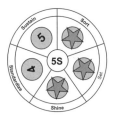

4th S Create and set **standards** for cleanliness.
Standardize to improve!

Standardize involves creating guidelines for keeping an area organized, orderly, and clean. This includes making those standards visual and obvious. The team and/or staff member would follow these steps:

 a. Identify the target area.
 b. Decide what the specific tasks are and where they should happen (location). List them on a sheet of paper.
 c. Decide who will perform the tasks. List in a column.
 d. Decide frequency and supplies required. List in a column and post in the target area.

5S Standards for Target Area				
Target Area _____				
Task	Location	Who	When	Supplies

 e. Create a Five Minute 5S Checklist (see next page).

Five Minute 5S Checklist

Team Members: _____

Purpose: To assist the team to complete assigned duties on time.

Target Area: _____   **Date:** _____

	Standard Time to Peform for _____(Ex. John)
SORT	Ex. John will put away extra supplies each day from OR 1 (1 minute).
SET-IN-ORDER	Ex. John will verify supply cabinets are stocked properly at start of day (1 minute).
SHINE	Ex. John will wipe down counters in exam room 2 after last patient (1 minute).
STANDARDIZE	Ex. John will walk through OR and determine if equipment is stored in correct location (1 minute).
SUSTAIN	Ex. John will sign-off on completing the Five Minute 5S Checklist.

f. Post appropriate forms in the target area.

g. Post the 5S visual circle in a common area and place a seal on the fourth S.

You may wish to rotate cleaning assignments weekly or monthly.

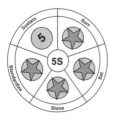

5th S Educate and communicate to ensure cleanliness is **sustained** over time.
   Sustain the gains!

The essence of Sustain is found in the saying, "Sustain all gains through self-discipline." This S will allow all staff to be trained in the 5S methodology. A learning environment must be created to support those participants who have attended the training sessions. This is vital because the information presented in these sessions must be linked directly to the staff's jobs.

The team and/or staff member would follow these steps:

a. Create the 5S Training Matrix. Training items are specific topics that require training (e.g., understanding the need, conducting audits, ordering supplies, etc.).

5S Training Matrix						
Name _____ Job Title _____ Dept _____						
Training Item	Sort	Set	Shine	Std	Sustain	Date

b. Regularly conduct the 5S Area Audit. (See next page.)

An audit will ensure standards are maintained once they have been created. After completion of the 5th S, brainstorm with the team to determine ways to energize the 5S process (visuals, rewards, office/unit/ward competitions, showcases, etc.) to maintain the momentum.

5S Area Audit

Auditor(s) _____

Work Area _____

5 or more problems, enter 0
3 or 4 problems, enter 1
2 problems, enter 2
1 problem, enter 3
0 problems, enter 4

Category	Activity	Date ___	Date ___	Date ___
Sort	1. Unneeded books, supplies, etc.			
	2. Unneeded reference materials, etc.			
	3. Items present in aisles, hallways, etc.			
	4. Safety concerns			
Set-In-Order	5. Correct places for items			
	6. Items are not put away			
	7. Work areas properly defined			
	8. Office equipment locations defined			
Shine	9. Desk surfaces and cabinets free of dust			
	10. Computer terminal screens clean			
	11. Cleaning materials easily accessible			
	12. Common areas looking clean			
	13. Labels, signs, etc. are clear to see			
Standardize	14. Work information is visible			
	15. 5S Standards are posted			
	16. Everyone trained to standards			
	17. Checklists exist for all areas			
	18. Items in areas can be located quickly			
Sustain	19. An audit sheet has been created			
	20. Audits are conducted regularly			
	21. Improvement ideas for 5S are used			

Healthcare facilities are like living organisms in that they change and grow. 5S must be a process that adapts as staff comes and goes, business conditions change, and new technology develops. 5S is the **foundation** for Lean healthcare.

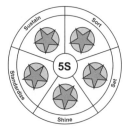

The benefits of 5S are:

- Provides the foundation for a Lean healthcare facility
- Assists in the elimination of waste
- Improves work flow
- Reduces employee stress
- Provides a systematic process for continuous improvement
- Focuses on the process and not the person

The 5S system can be immediately applied to an entire department allowing everyone to get involved in the Lean process and activity.

Note: Many times an organization may add a 6th S of Safety and a 7th S of Spirit.

For detailed information, it is recommended you obtain *Lean Healthcare: 5 Keys to Improving the Healthcare Environment, The 5S for the Office User's Guide, and The 5S Desktop (PC) Pocket Handbook available* at http://www.theleanstore.com.

Key Points for 5S in Healthcare

- 5S must be part of everyone's daily work.
- Make sure the first S "sort" is done well, as it will set the stage for the other S's.
- Ensure before and after photos are taken and displayed.
- Obtain testimonials from workers during the process and submit them to the facility newsletter.
- Be creative and adaptive to the changing healthcare environment.
- Make reward and recognition part of the process.

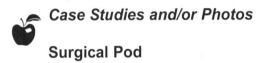

Case Studies and/or Photos

Surgical Pod

A hospital had constant complaints from the surgical doctors and nurses that numerous times a nurse or technician had to leave the operating room during the procedure to retrieve an item. Even though surgical supplies should have been on the cart or in the extra supply cabinet within the operating room, the additional item was missing. This frantic search for a supply caused stress for the entire surgical team - and extended the procedure time. A Lean 5S team was established to apply the principle of 5S to alleviate this situation. The following team members were gathered: a clinical manager, pod technician, endoscopy technician, scrub technician, and two operating room RNs. The team received training in 5S. The team focused on one pod (4 operating rooms), while meeting every two weeks (1 - 2 hours each time) throughout a three month period. This resulted in the following outcomes:

1) Saved over $1600 in surplus supplies found in the operating room's supply cabinet
2) Reduced time leaving the OR by 88%
3) Reduced stress on the surgical team

Radiology

The Radiology staff was motivated to implement 5S in their department after hearing the benefits of a successful team effort that had implemented 5S in their ED. They spent a week red-tagging the items not in use. They thought they would find a few items, but to their surprise, they found that almost 50% of the items in their storage area were no longer in use. These items were being kept "just-in-case," but no one could remember the last time they were actually used. The team decided to discard most of those items and sent a few to the warehouse with a review date of 6 months; if never needed, they would be discarded.

Once "Sort" was done, the "Set-In-Order" phase went quickly. With so much room freed up by the removal of old items, the team was able to move boxes and supplies out of hallways and off of countertops. "Shine Week" went well also, with most staff members pitching in. The Radiology Manager said the department had never looked so good! Patients made favorable comments as well. The team put together their standards and created an audit checklist for "Sustain."

The entire effort took only five weeks, roughly one week for each phase, and staff members agreed to rotate the responsibilities for the audit. 5S became a standing agenda item on the monthly department meeting. Soon, it seemed hard to remember what the department looked like before the 5S effort.

The results were as follows:
1) Increase of 300 square feet of floor space
2) $10,500 worth of equipment taken off the books as not needed or was not found

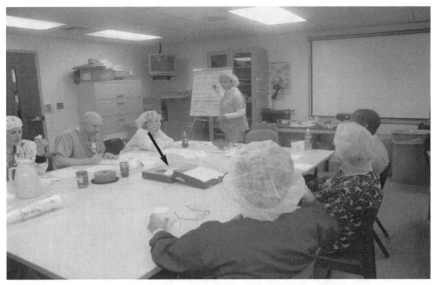

Staff members must come together and meet as a team and reach a consensus on the 5S projects. Donuts help!

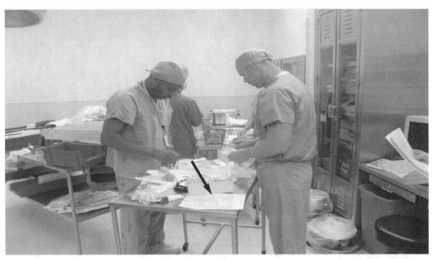

When conducting the Sort portion of 5S, have the Sort Inspection Sheet (or guidelines) nearby.

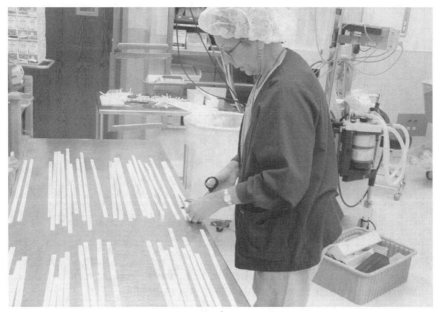

Labels are made one at a time for Set-In-Order. Do not underestimate the value in labeling items and locations.

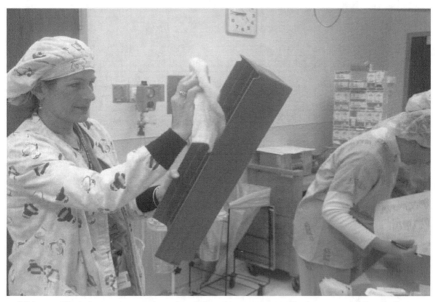

Shine will get everyone involved to clean areas that may not have been cleaned in quite a while.

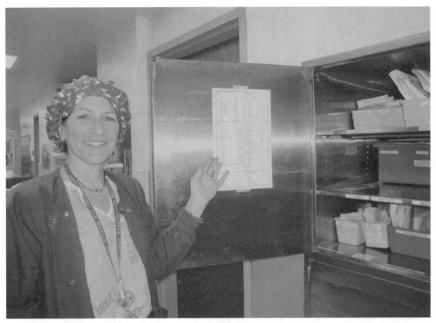

Standard involves creating the guidelines for keeping an area organized and cleaned.

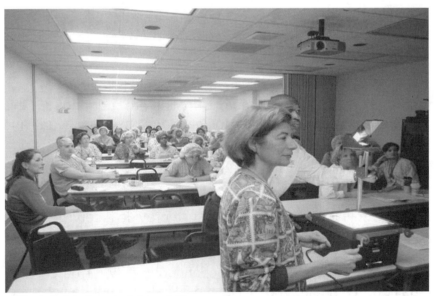

Sustain involves training staff so everyone can fully understand the 5S program and what it means for the organization.

Continuous Flow

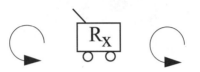

 Why use it?

Continuous flow is used to move work, patients, or provide a service between processes with minimal or no wait time.

Who does it?

A Lean team will be established to review current work and/or patient flow. The Lean team will brainstorm to see how physical layout, cross-training, and eliminating waste can improve this movement.

How long will it take?

Depending on your area, this process could take hours or days as furniture, equipment, and/or supplies are rearranged. This will be an ongoing activity to maintain improved work and patient flow.

What does it do?

Continuous flow is the ability to provide a service or item when requested. (See Just-In-Time)

There are various degrees of continuous flow. True continuous flow in a healthcare facility most likely will not be achieved. Therefore, the tools of In-process supermarkets and FIFO lanes can be utilized to assist work flow. These will be defined on the following pages.

In-Process Supermarkets (or areas of supply replenishment)

The In-process supermarket (i.e., the grocery store shelf between the supplier of the goods and the consumer) exists due to the variations in customer demand. The customer's lead time is minimal (the time it takes to remove something off the shelf), therefore, it would not be feasible to have just one item there. In order to establish the In-process supermarket, an ordering pattern, establishing minimum and maximum levels needs to be determined to create a balance between what the customer demand is and the frequency of delivery to the store (and shelf). In-process supermarkets can also be explained in terms of cycle time. A supermarket exists between two processes to accommodate the differences in the cycle times of those processes (i.e., the time for the removal of a grocery item from the store shelf to the time it takes to replenish those items from the warehouse). This is called the pull system. Only the amount that has been used by the customer for that day, week, or month (depending on the ordering pattern), or "pulled" from the shelf, is reordered. The maximum level is never exceeded.

For In-process supermarkets to be successful, the following will need to be in place:

- A quantitative understanding of the downstream requirements
- Known cycle times for the downstream and upstream processes
- Communication system between the upstream and downstream processes
- Minimum and maximum number of work units or service capacity assigned to the supermarket
- A signal or "kanban" triggers a "pull" from the downstream process to replenish what was removed

For example, supplies in many healthcare departments can run out on a hourly, daily, or weekly basis. To minimize this disruption and maintain optimal care for the patient, In-process supermarkets for unit/floor supply areas may provide value. The supermarkets would limit extra supplies throughout the area and prevent the searching for needed supplies at critical times. The supplies at these locations would be located in an In-process supermarket, meeting the hourly and daily needs of the staff. Replenishment of the supplies would be through kanban cards when supplies reached a minimum ordering level.

It should be noted that information (i.e., charts, labs, consults, etc.) can also be considered a "supply" or "supermarket item" and the supermarket concept can be applied as such.

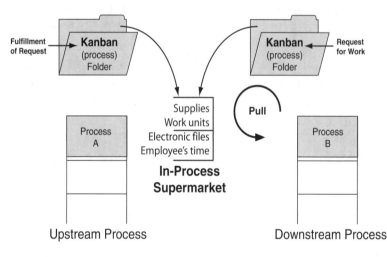

First-In First-Out Lanes (or FIFO Lanes)

Another way to control the flow between processes is a method referred to as First-In First-Out or (FIFO). FIFO is a work controlled method to ensure the oldest work upstream (first-in) is the first to be processed downstream (first-out).

For example, in central supply areas, sterile materials are continuously rotated to replace the materials with the up and coming expiration date at the front of the shelf. This can also apply to work requests in pharmacy, pathology, radiology, medical records, etc.

The FIFO lane has the following attributes:

- Located between two processes
- A maximum number of work units (materials, meds, etc.) are placed in the FIFO lane and are visible
- Is sequentially loaded and labeled
- Has a signal system to notify the upstream process when the lane is full
- Has visual rules and standards posted to ensure FIFO lane integrity
- Has a process in place for assisting the downstream process when the lane is full and assistance is required

The team can be creative in establishing the signal method within the FIFO system to indicate when the system is full. This could be a raised flag, a light, a pager code, a text message, or an urgent email to the upstream process. The important point is to ensure a signal is established that will work effectively. When the signal is released, the upstream worker lends support to the downstream worker until the work is caught up. There is no point in continuing to produce upstream when the downstream process is overloaded. When this happens, it becomes an overproduction waste, which is considered the worst waste of all.

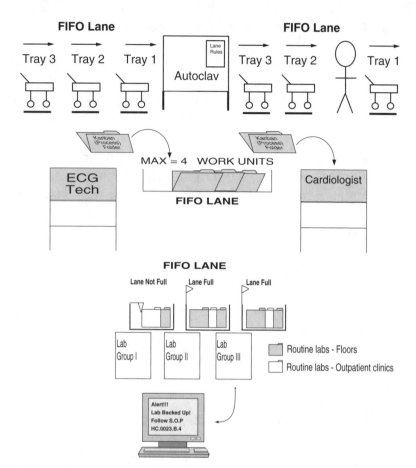

The benefits of In-process supermarkets and FIFO lanes are:

- Reduction in overall lead times (preparation times)
- Reduction in wait times
- Easier identification and rectification of problems when they occur
- Increased process efficiency and throughput
- Reduction of stress

How do you do it?

There are seven steps in determining how to improve the area for continuous flow.

1. Review the current office arrangement and process tasks. Determine which wastes are involved in terms of travel, motion, and lack of cross-training.

2. Brainstorm with the team to consolidate office arrangements to reduce or eliminate the wastes identified in step 1. Processes may need to be modified or standardized. People may need to be trained to understand this new process.

3. Determine if an In-process supermarket or FIFO lane is required.

4. Prepare a plan to implement proposed changes with expected results. Make sure to obtain management approval.

5. Implement the new layout and/or new process(es).

6. Balance the work loads among staff members. (See Work Load Balancing)

7. Consider new technologies and software enhancements as you continue to improve.

Key Points for Continuous Flow in Healthcare

- Both the In-process supermarket and FIFO lanes are compromises to pure continuous flow.
- In-process supermarkets are more commonly used for office and medical supplies.
- FIFO lanes are the most common tool to improve administrative work and patient flow.
- Intensive cross-training and work standardization are great tools to assist continuous flow.

Case Studies and/or Photos

Outpatient Laboratory Department

The staff of an outpatient laboratory department used the concept of continuous flow to improve the outpatient specimen collection process. In examining the old process, the team found that after signing-in, every patient sat down in the waiting room to wait. The wait time averaged 16 minutes. After creating and identifying this waiting waste on a value stream map, the staff of the outpatient lab changed this procedure. Now, more than 90% of patients never have to wait in the waiting room. Patients are immediately taken to a drawing chair instead. The staff created a First-In First-Out (FIFO) lane. If more than three people are on the list to have blood drawn, a second phlebotomist is called (via a visual cue) to help. Patient waiting time is thereby reduced to a minimum. An additional improvement was realized through further analysis of the future state value stream map. This was a reduction in the time involved in delivering specimens from the outpatient area to the processing area by adding more lab pick-ups. This resulted in the following outcomes:

1. Increased patient satisfaction because of decreased waiting times
2. Decreased time to obtain lab results

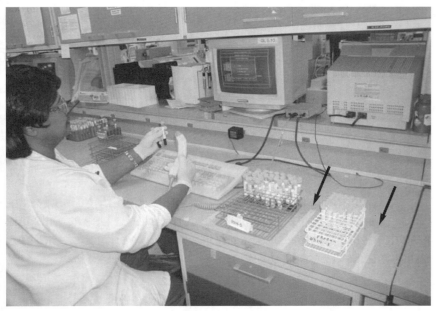

FIFO lanes do not have to be difficult to implement, sometimes masking tape can work just fine.

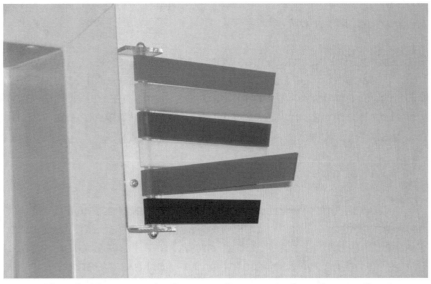

Visual aids can assist the overall concept of continuous flow.

Cycle Time

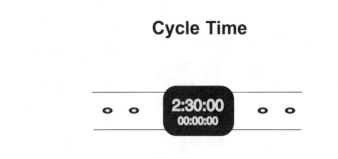

Why use it?

This tool establishes the time elapsed from the beginning of a work process until it is completed. Use it with takt time to establish the best combination of work load and task assignments. (See Takt Time)

Who does it?

Anyone familiar with the processes or tasks will use it.

How long will it take?

Processes (tasks, activities, procedures) can take anywhere from 3 seconds (i.e., a computer entry) to several weeks (i.e., following a physician's referral form from beginning to end). Establishing accurate times for each of the steps in the process is critical.

What does it do?

Cycle time is the amount of time required for a task to be completed. This should not be confused with takt time. Cycle time is the rate of the process. It allows for a clear understanding of the number of workers needed for the process, task, or value stream (if takt time is known). Cycle time (as well as takt time) should be used with standard work. (See Standard Work)

There are three types of cycle times:

Individual cycle time is the rate of completion of an individual task or single operation of work. For example, entering patient data into the Electronic Medical Records system.

Total cycle time is the rate of completion of a process or group of tasks that have a common element. This is calculated by adding up the individual cycle times for that process. For example, preparing a patient to be seen by a healthcare provider will require the following tasks: obtain history of visit, height, weight, and vital sign measurements, etc., each having separate cycle times. The total cycle time would be the summation of all those activities related to preparing the patient for the exam.

Group cycle time is the rate of completing a group task or objective. This is the total individuals' times added together for a project. For example, tracking an emergency room admission from entry into the Emergency Room through hospital admission and/or discharge would be comprised of many processes and departments. The summation of these process cycle times would equal a group cycle time.

 How do you do it?

There are four steps in determining how to use cycle times for increased efficiencies.

1. Individual cycle times are obtained by adding all steps (or individual tasks) for a process.

Cycle Time Table

Staff - Unit Coordinator			Staff - Nurse			Staff - Doctor		
Step	Description	Cycle Time	Step	Description	Cycle Time	Step	Description	Cycle Time
1	Chart Retrieval	3 min	1	Hx of patient	2 min	1	Review chart	2 min
2	Enter patient data	3 min	2	Reports to Dr.	3 min	2	Patient questions	2 min
3	Referral to Specialist	10 min	3	Follow-up w/ patient	10 min	3	Exam	5 min
Total Time		16 min			15 min			9 min

2. Add the individual cycle times to obtain the total cycle time for the various steps.

	Unit Coord.	Nurse	Doctor
Total Cycle time =	16 min +	15 min +	9 min

= 40 minutes total cycle time

3. Calculate takt time. You calculate takt time by dividing the available work time for a day (minus meetings, breaks, etc.) by the total volume of work required for that day. (See Takt Time)

Typical day for first shift in a facility:

7:00 – 7:10	morning meeting – not available work time	
7:10 – 9:30	available work time	**140 min**
9:30 – 9:40	morning break – not available work time	
9:40 – 11:00	available work time	**80 min**
11:00 – 12:00	lunch – not available work time	
12:00 – 2:00	available work time	**120 min**
2:00 – 2:10	afternoon break – not available work time	
2:10 – 2:40	meetings (average this for the week) – not available work time	
2:40 – 4:00	available work time	**80 min**

Total available work time is:

140 m + 80 m + 120 m + 80 m = 420 minutes per day (m=minutes)

Let us say the volume of work is 30 patients per day.

$$\frac{420 \text{ minutes per day}}{30 \text{ patients per day}} = 14 \text{ minute takt time}$$

4. Dividing the total cycle time by the takt time will determine the total number of staff required for the tasks.

Optimal number of staff required =

$$\frac{40 \text{ minutes (total cycle time)}}{14 \text{ minutes (takt time)}} = 2.86 \text{ staff (or 3 staff to meet the demand for that process)}$$

Healthcare has a version of this already in existence. For example, on a med-surg floor, if the census is above the determined limit, an extra staff member is called in.

Key Points for Cycle Time in Healthcare

- It may be a challenge to obtain cycle times, but do not let that stop you. Even though the times may not be as accurate as they should be, at least start to establish them. You will always be coming back to these times in kaizen activities. (See Kaizen Events)
- When determining the optimal number of staff needed:
    - If decimal is greater than or equal to .5, round up
    - If decimal is less than .5, round down (and kaizen to possibly use staff in another area that has a need)
- Kaizen is used to eliminate, reduce, and streamline the individual cycle times. Do not use this as a tool to reduce staff in the facility.
- It is suggested that multiple cycle times be collected to determine the most accurate number representing that particular process or task time.

Case Studies and/or Photos

Radiology

CT scanning (Computed or Computerized Tomography) is a valuable diagnostic tool. CTs are taken from a series of different angles and are arranged by a computer to show a cross-sectional view of organs in the body. CT scanning provides significantly more detailed information than X-rays.

One hospital's CT technicians used Lean to improve their CT scanning processes. Since CT scans have become a diagnostic tool of choice, the demand for CT scans has increased dramatically. Because CT scanning equipment is expensive, and CT technicians are in short supply, hospital administrators cannot simply purchase more CT machines or hire more technicians. In this hospital, a Lean team was formed. Cycle time observations via data capture and process mapping showed that CT technicians were obtaining patient data and prepping the patient while in the CT scan room. This was a waste of scan time, machine availability, and the technician's technical training.

The technicians changed the information gathering process so that support personnel would complete the patient preparation process before positioning the patient on the CT equipment. This resulted in the following outcomes:

1. Decreased cycle time of the CT scan per patient
2. Increased CT equipment usage for scans
3. Two CT technicians were assigned to fill other open positions

Document Tagging

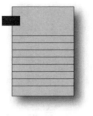

 Why use it?

This tool accurately captures the amount of time it takes for a chart, document, or patient to travel through a process, area, or value stream.

Who does it?

A core team will work to determine the process(es) or value stream to be tagged. Everyone connected to the process will contribute and document their time.

How long does it take?

This will take only a few seconds to a few minutes a day to accomplish.

 What does it do?

This allows the Lean healthcare team to collect the necessary data on the various cycle times and value-added work. Document tagging accomplishes the following:

* Continues to create awareness of organizational time
* Involves everyone connected to the process
* Once complete, analysis of the process will be based on actual times - not estimates
* Provides data for creating an accurate current state value stream map (See Value Stream Mapping)

How do you do it?

1. Determine the process(es) or value stream on which data will be collected.

2. Create the Document Tagging Worksheet in Microsoft Word or Excel and label the various columns.

		In		Out			Time in Minutes				
Step	**Name/Dept.**	Date	Time	Date	Time	**Task/Activity**	Delay/Wait Time from Previous Step	Cycle Time	Elapsed Time	Value-Added Time	Non Value-Added Time
1											
2											
3											
4											
5											
6											
7											
8											
9											
10											
11											
12											
13											
14											
15											
16											
						TOTALS					

Document Tagging Worksheet

Value Stream _____ Start Date In _____
Process _____ Start Date Out _____

Notes:
Delay/Wait Time is calculated by subtracting the In Time from the Out Time of the previous step.
Cycle Time is calculated by subtracting the beginning time of the step from the end time of the step.
Elapsed Time is the Delay/Wait Time plus the Cycle Time accumulated from each step (running total).
Value-Added Time is the time required to physically (or electronically) transform the service into value for the patient or customer (other healthcare provider or department). It typically is the cycle time minus any delay or wait time for that step.
Non Value-Added Time is calculated by adding the Delay/Wait Time plus any Cycle Time that does not add value to the patient (or customer).

Analysis:

3. Communicate to the group what information is required on the form (you may need to refresh the group with information from the Business Case for Lean Healthcare section). Ensure the tasks are described as a verb-noun combination (e.g., assemble equipment, verbally prepare the patient, prepare arm, draw blood, etc.).

4. Distribute the form to the most upstream process in the value stream. This will be where the work or patient originates. This is like placing an "alert" or tag on a document (e.g., patient chart) and following it through the various processes until it reaches the most downstream process.

5. Collect all of the data. Do this four or five times to ensure accuracy. The staff are required to document the following columns:

> Step – this should be sequential
> Name/Dept
> Date
> Time In
> Date
> Time Out
> Task/Activity
> Cycle Time

6. Utilize data to establish the best cycle time for the process(es). Once the document has reached the final process, the following information should be analyzed:

Delay/Wait Time: Subtract In Time from the Out Time of the previous step
Cycle Time: Subtract the beginning time of the step from the end time of the step
Elapsed Time: Add Delay/Wait Time to Cycle Time
Value-Added Time: This is the time required to physically (or electronically) transform the service into value for the patient or customer (other healthcare provider or department). It typically is the cycle time minus any delay or wait time for that step.
Non Value-Added Time: Add the Delay/Wait Time to any cycle time that does not add value (i.e., additional wait time)

7. Create the Standard Work Chart. Use this as a basis for improvement activities. (See Standard Work)

8. Train staff on the new standard and update the Process Master Document. (See Paper File System)

Document Tagging Worksheet

Value Stream Dispo-to-Admit   **Start Date In** 4/10

Process ED Dispo to Chart Prep   **Start Date Out** 4/10

		In		Out			Time in Minutes				
Step	Name/Dept.	Date	Time	Date	Time	Task/Activity	Delay/Wait Time from Previous Step	Cycle Time	Elapsed Time	Value-Added Time	Non Value-Added Time
1	Doctor	4/10	0823	4/10	0833	Write Dispo/Admit Order	0	10	10	10	0
2	Doctor	4/10	0833	4/10	0838	Perform medication reconciliation	0	5	15	5	0
3	Doctor	4/10	0840	4/10	0841	Not Dispo (Admit) Order in chart	2	1	18	0	3
4	ED Clerk	4/10	0857	4/10	0859	Process Admit Order in IT system	16	2	36	0	18
5	ED Clerk	4/10	0907	4/10	0908	Place face sheet in chart	8	1	45	0	9
6	ED Clerk	4/10	0912	4/10	0925	Copy ED chart for IP chart	4	13	62	0	17
7	ED Nurse	4/10	0932	4/10	0936	Complete Med/Allergy form	7	4	73	4	7
8	ED Nurse	4/10	0936	4/10	0946	Complete charting record for IP unit	0	10	83	10	0
9	ED Nurse	4/10	0946	4/10	0949	Refer to chart when IP unit is called	0	3	86	3	0
10	ED Tech	4/10	0952	4/10	0955	Complete clothing check form in chart	3	3	92	0	6
11	ED Tech	4/10	0957	4/10	0958	Note vital signs in chart	2	1	95	1	2
12	ED Tech	4/10	1001	4/10	1004	Call transporter, note in chart	3	3	101	0	6
13	ED Nurse	4/10	1007	4/10	1010	Note last vital signs	3	3	107	3	3
14	ED Clerk	4/10	1012	4/10	1014	Place chart, face sheet, wst band, und. matt.	2	2	111	0	4
15	ED Nurse	4/10	1019	4/10	1020	Note call to IP Ns. Mgr. when patient leaves	5	1	117	0	6
16	Transporter	4/10	1023	4/10	1024	Check chart is ready to travel w/ patient	3	1	121	0	4
						TOTALS	58	63	121	36	85

Notes:
Delay/Wait Time is calculated by subtracting the In Time from the Out Time of the previous step.
Cycle Time is calculated by subtracting the beginning time of the step from the end time of the step.
Elapsed Time is the Delay/Wait Time plus the Cycle Time accumulated from each step (running total).
Value-Added Time is the time required to physically (or electronically) transform the service into value for the patient or customer (other healthcare provider or department). It typically is the cycle time minus any delay or wait time for that step.
Non Value-Added Time is calculated by adding the Delay/Wait Time plus any Cycle Time that does not add value to the patient (or customer).

Analysis:
Total chart activity time, from Dispo written to patient leaving, was 121 minutes or 2 hours, 1 minute (from 0823 to 1024). Note: this is less than the 170 minutes total lead time for the Dispo-to-Admit value stream because the Document Tagging ends when the patient leaves the ED.
The value-added time was 36 minutes.
Therefore, the chart was being used approximately 30% of the time, with the other 70% of the time being inactive.
This demonstrated the amount of information that must be ready prior to the patient being transferred to the inpatient bed from the ED. More importantly, it validated much of the information from the Cycle Time Table and other data collection tools used to create the current state value stream map. It also provided additional insight (and possible solutions) to the delays that were occurring.
This information was used to provide more detail to the current state value stream map. *It will not match exactly the Cycle Time Table because the focus of this data was the chart information process.*

Key Points for Document Tagging in Healthcare

- Imagine an "alert" or tag on a document as the document proceeds through the value stream.
- Communicate to employees that the focus is waste in the process. This "tagging activity" will assist in identifying it.
- After tagging is completed, a process map or value stream map can be created with more accuracy.
- Even though facility processes are unique, many will have similarities in functions. If you capture 80% of common work tasks in a process, utilize that as the foundation for improvement.
- Consider color-coding documents if multiple value streams are being analyzed at once.

Error Proofing

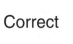 Correct Incorrect

 Why use it?

This applies error or mistake prevention into a process to achieve zero defects. It is also known as Poka-Yoke or Mistake-Proofing.

Who does it?

The project team that is experienced in Lean will incorporate error proofing where it is feasible.

How long does it take?

It will take brainstorming, testing ideas, and further data collection to determine the best error proofing techniques. This can be accomplished in a few hours, but may take more time to implement and verify effectiveness.

 What does it do?

This tool specifically addresses processes that generate mistakes (i.e., billing, medical records, scheduling, etc.). Error proofing accomplishes the following:

- Improves quality of patient care and service
- Corrects conditions in the process that allow for errors or mistakes
- Supports ideas from knowledgeable staff to improve a process or area
- Reduces costs to the organization by eliminating duplication of work

How do you do it?

The aim of error proofing is to attain a level of Lean sophistication so errors that may produce defects are not generated. Defects and errors are not the same thing.

Defects vs. Errors

To be a defect:

- The process or service must have deviated from specifications or standards of service

- The process or service does not meet customer (internal or external) expectations

To be an error:

- Something must have deviated from an intended process

- All defects are created by errors, but not all errors result in defects

---

The five steps to error proofing are:

1. Shift your paradigm.
2. Conduct analysis.
3. Standardize the work.
4. Create "alert" conditions.
5. Create error proofing devices or systems.

1. Shift your paradigm.

Errors can be prevented! Begin looking for the source of defects, not just the defects themselves. At the same time look for opportunities to eliminate them at their source. Everyone must understand that they are playing by a new set of rules. The root cause of defects is in the process, not the people.

---

2. Conduct analysis.

To analyze the problem you must be able to identify and describe the defect or potential error in depth, including the rate it may have been occurring over time. A Failure Prevention Analysis Worksheet (FPAW) can assist in this process. Failure Prevention Analysis is a technique that allows the team to anticipate potential problems in the solution before implementing it. This allows the team to be proactive to prevent the solution(s) from going wrong. The subsequent processes of mistake proofing would be the procedures, visual controls, alarm notifications, etc. that would prevent a mistake from being made or to ensure the mistake, if made, is obvious at a glance.

The following guidelines will assist you in using the Failure Prevention Analysis Worksheet:

a. Create a list of potential failures for each improvement activity that has a probable cause-effect relationship with an opportunity for error.
b. Rank the potential failures by rating the potential and consequence for each possibility for each item going wrong on a scale from 1 to 10.
c. Multiply the potential and consequence together for each of the potential failures (1) to give the overall rating.
d. Rank each potential failure from highest to lowest (1 - XX).
e. Brainstorm with the team to modify any/all activities to lessen the likelihood of causing a problem.
f. Continue with the improvement project.

The following illustration is an example of a Failure Prevention Analysis Worksheet.

Failure Prevention Analysis Worksheet

Directions:
1. List all potential failures.
2. Assign a number from 1 to 5 for the potential and consequence of an activity going wrong.
3. Multiply the potential and consequence and rank from highest to lowest.

Potential Rating

1 - Very unlikely to occur - once a year
2 - Might occur rarely - once a month
3 - 50/50 chance to occur within five days
4 - Good chance to occur at least once a day
5 - Excellent chance to occur several times a day

Consequence Rating

1 - Very little or no risk to the patient
2 - Some risk to the patient, but easily corrected
3 - Moderate risk to the patient, needing some action
4 - Severe risk to the patient, requiring action
5 - Most severe consequence to the patient, possible
    death, requiring immediate action

Potential Failure	Potential	Consequence	Overall Rating	Ranking
A. Physicians can't reach PCP for consult (after 15 min. from first call)	3	1	3	5
B. Clerk doesn't see dispo in chart, even though Dr. places it there	1	4	4	4
C. Pt belongings missing, even though form used when pt was in ED	2	4	8	3
D. Quick Reg page prints but is not seen; printer is dedicated	3	4	12	2
E. Transporter still busy with other patients when called for by ED	3	5	15	1

Improvement Solutions:

A. The ED physician would continue with patient care (and admit process) without waiting for PCP call back. When (and if) the PCP would call back at that time the ED physician would discuss patient care.
B. The team asked the computer support group to investigate whether they could "broadcast" a message to all registrars computer terminals that an ED Admit had been ordered, to assure that the registrars would know that an admit order needed to be processed.
C. The team discussed the possibility that the patient might have additional items of value, besides clothing, that were not noted at the time the form was started; for example, a necklace that was not removed initially, but was then removed for an X-ray. The team decided that training was needed for all staff that came in contact with the patient and the belongings form needed to travel with the patient rather than being placed in the chart.
D. A separate printer had been placed in the Registration area to handle admitting requests from the ED. However, there was still a possibility that a busy registrars might not see the forms immediately, and the audible signal (B) might not be heard in a busy environment.
E. The team added to the unit reporting form a checkbox for transporter being called to remind the Nurse to do that right away. Earlier notification would help the transporter prioritize the work. The team had also piloted the use of a dedicated elevator, which did not seem to be a significant factor at this time, so they discontinued that trial.

There are two points in a Lean project where the FPAW may be useful: (1) when developing the solutions, the FPAW can help the team to determine whether any of the proposed solutions may cause unforeseen consequences; and (2), after solutions have been implemented, to determine whether some activities happen with more frequency or more severe consequences than anticipated.

The FPAW is most useful:

- When studying the current process, the FPAW can be used to point out the most problematic areas of the current state and which problems would be the most important to fix.
- When developing the future state, the FPAW can be used to imagine what problems might occur if the process were changed.
- When reviewing the standard work after the change has been implemented, the FPAW can be used to analyze the mistakes and problems that are apparent based on observation and feedback.

3. Standardize the work.

Create standard work instructions and communicate to any staff that does not follow the standards. The standard can be written documentation already in existence (i.e, policy manuals, service standards, work instructions, etc.). Obtain a consensus on all new standard work procedures to eliminate any opportunities for error. (See Standard Work)

4. Create "alert" conditions.

Use visual controls as much as possible to identify conditions that may cause an error. (See Visual Controls)

5. Create error proofing devices or systems.

There are three levels of control that error proofing devices can achieve:

Level 1 - Indicators - providing information about the immediate environment, area, department or process. These are passive and people may or may not notice them or respond to them. A Level 1 visual control may be a sign displaying the "Triple Check" procedure for dispersing medications. Another example would be ensuring "Allergy Alert" is highlighted in red on the patient's chart and ID bracelet.

Level 2 - Signals - causing a visual or auditory alarm that should grab your attention and is a warning that a mistake or error is about to occur. People still may ignore these, but they are very aware that something may be wrong. A Level 2 visual control may be typing in the patient's medications on the computer and a visual or auditory alert would occur if there was a potential for a drug interaction. If codeine is ordered for a patient, and the patient is allergic to codeine, the pharmacy computer program would issue "med/alert" on the computer screen.

Level 3 - Physical or Electronic Controls - limiting or preventing something from occurring due to its negative impact it will have on the process (or area) (most likely referred to as mistake proofing devices). A Level 3 visual control may be the mechanical wall connections for medical gases, such as oxygen and nitrogen. Each of these devices has access ports that will only fit the appropriate gas, oxygen for oxygen and nitrogen for nitrogen.

Clearly Level 3 is most desirable, but not always possible or cost effective.

Key Points for Error Proofing in Healthcare

- The goal of error proofing is zero defects.
- All staff must understand the importance of error proofing ar believe that *any error* can be prevented.
- Error proofing reduces cycle times and prevents wastes su as: waiting, transporting, errors, etc.
- Always focus on the process and not the staff.

Case Studies and/or Photos

Nosocomial Infections

"Stop-the-line" was implemented in a hospital's Critical Care U (CCU) when the number of bloodstream infections increased. root cause analysis was performed and showed that the caus of the infections were due to staff and physicians not washi their hands consistently and not following the evidence-bas best practices for the care of central lines. The hospital launch a hand washing campaign for the consistent use of the guidelin of central lines. As a result, the bloodstream infection rate w decreased and remained at or near 0%. The unit also went eic months with no incidents of ventilator-acquired pneumonia. Th resulted in the following outcomes:

1. Decreased nosocomial infection rate
2. Decreased costs from eliminating the need to treat nosoc mial infections
3. Provided safer patient care
4. Increased staff satisfaction through empowerment to "stc the-line"

Pharmacy

The hospital had introduced an automated-delivery system for medications. Each nursing unit had a dispensing module that was run by the hospital's computer system and linked into the Pharmacy Information System. Pharmacy would stock the dispensing module with medications that had been ordered for patients on that unit. To obtain the medication, the nurse entered the patient's account number, then the correct drawer would open and the nurse could retrieve the meds.

However, as a precaution against a possible emergency need, the nurses had been given a password to access the module without a specific patient account number. Over time, nurses found it easier to use the password than to bring the account number with them in the form of a chart, patient form, or note. Eventually, almost 25% of the withdrawals were being done via that password, rather than specific account numbers. The nurses did not see any difference, but the non-specific password made it impossible for the medication billing to be processed correctly, and also had an impact on the accuracy of the electronic Medication Administration Record (MAR).

The Pharmacy studied the number of times withdrawals were made in actual emergency situations and concluded that there had been none since the inception of the dispensing module. They believed that there should still be an override function, but they limited that to the Nursing leaders on the unit (via their ID badge bar code) and changed the programming of the module to allow only patient-specific account numbers to be used for withdrawals. They performed in-service training to all of the nurses, pointing out the advantages of an accurate MAR (which meant less work in the daily reconciliation that was performed). The percentage of over-ride withdrawals after this change was less than 2%.

Lab

When blood specimens were ordered and collected by non-lab personnel, the bar-code labels were printed on the nursing units. Unfortunately, to be read by lab instrumentation bar-code readers, the labels had to be placed a certain way on the tube. There were numerous times that the labels had to be reprinted and replaced on the tubes which caused delays in getting the test results. The lab team brainstormed ways to resolve the issue, and then worked with their Lab Information System staff to add a small arrow with the word "UP" on the label. The team then in-serviced all the nursing units that the arrow needed to point toward the cap. In this way, they reduced the number of "defective" labels (which had to be removed and replaced before testing) from 45% to 7% within two weeks.

Goals and Outcomes

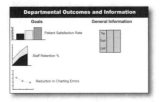

 Why use it?

Appropriate short and long term goals and measurements can verify the impact on improvement activities.

Who does it?

The Lean project team will establish goals and outcomes consistent with the strategic direction. Staff will contribute by working towards their individual and/or team goals.

How long does it take?

Establishing goals and expected outcomes may take a few hours. The time may vary depending on whether staff are working on individual or team goals.

 What does it do?

Goals will focus on outcomes. Outcomes will be the result of reducing and eliminating wastes. Goals will also:

- Assess individual/team performance
- Establish a baseline goal on which to improve
- Establish outcomes
- Improve the facility's overall efficiency by improving team and/or individual goals

How do you do it?

There are seven steps in developing and implementing Lean Healthcare goals.

1. Review Team Charter for strategic direction.
2. Establish Lean goals.
3. Obtain a consensus for goals.
4. Calculate baseline goals.
5. Select outcomes.
6. Create visual aid(s).
7. Measure and post results.

1. Review Team Charter for strategic direction.

Review the Team Charter to ensure a thorough understanding of what needs to be measured. The Team Charter should work to benefit the facility.

2. Establish Lean goals.

Goals are based on eliminating wastes. To find the goals that best fit your value stream, brainstorm with the team and gain a consensus. Some examples of goals are:

- Reduction in invoicing, requisition, or charting errors
- Reduction in patient or staff complaints
- Improvement in patient wait times while in the system
- Improvement in project completion percentages
- Improvement in staff retention rates and job satisfaction
- Individual productivity improvements
- Improvement in patient satisfaction

Goals established must be something the group, department, or individual has control over. (See Goal Card)

3. Obtain a consensus for goals.

Once the team has established the goals, they should be reviewed by management. This is required because resources may need to be allocated. Use the catchball process between the team and management to reach an agreement on the goals. In this process, the team members and managers "toss" ideas and proposals back and forth, refining them until a consensus is reached.

4. Calculate baseline goals.

Collect initial measurements to determine the starting point or baseline. Decide on the following:

- Who will be responsible for each goal
- How often it will be measured
- The type of form on which the information will be reported and to whom it will be reported
- The type of visual aid and where it will be displayed

The following worksheet can be utilized in organizing the proposed goals.

Goal Planning Worksheet

1. Decide which goals you will use, then enter them in the worksheet below.
2. Work from left to right for each goal. Do not skip any part!
3. Gain consensus on goals from management.

Goal	Who is Responsible	How Often Measured	Form Used to Measure	To Whom to Report	Visual Display Location

5. Select outcomes.

Do not forget to perform the back and forth process (i.e., catch-ball) again to ensure goals are reasonable and doable.

6. Create visual aid(s).

Outcomes, as well as goals, that are not made visual, will fail! Post these measurements (and goals) where they can be easily viewed. Posting these will create buy-in.

7. Measure and post results.

Create a schedule to ensure all departmental goals are updated on a regular basis. Departmental goals should be updated on a monthly, if not weekly basis. Individual or team goals should be updated on a weekly, if not daily, basis.

Key Points for Goals and Outcomes in Healthcare

- Use catchball to ensure goals are in alignment with management.
- Goals provide a total measure for the entire value stream, as well as specific outcomes for individual areas.
- Create a process for reviewing and updating the posted goals.
- Consider using graphs, not just numbers. Graphs are easier to read and understand. They communicate more effectively than words or numbers.
- Ensure recognition and rewards are in place for met outcomes.
- You cannot manage what cannot be measured.
- Finally, you treasure what you measure.

Goal Card

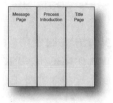

 Why use it?

This ensures that the strategic direction of the facility is embraced by all staff. This visual aid in pamphlet form encompasses Lean and/or Six Sigma healthcare vision and goals.

Who does it?

Top management will create the strategic direction. Managers, supervisors, and staff will contribute to what their support will be in terms of measurable outcomes.

How long will it take?

The strategic plan usually takes 1-2 days at an off-site meeting. The involvement of the entire facility, along with creating the Goal Cards, usually takes 1-2 months.

What does it do?

The Goal Card is the end result of a process that unites the facility's goals (strategic direction) with department and individual goals. It is the first step in Total Employee Involvement. Only by involving everyone – those who know their job the best – will a facility achieve its goals. It will be the individuals contributing to this process who will make the difference.

Overall Design

A typical Goal Card measures 8" x 11" and is made of card stock. It is folded into three sections, allowing for six panels on which to display information as shown in the illustration below.

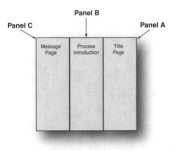

Management prepares the three exterior panels. Panel A is the front of the card when folded and acts as the title page. Panel B introduces the process of the Goal Card and is usually written by the senior manager in the organization. Panel C is the back page and will contain references to the strategic plan and is written by the President, CEO, and/or COO of the organization.

Departmental team members will gain a consensus and prepare the three interior panels. Panel D will contain the facilities' or Systems' strategy and goals (Level I). Panel E will convey the Lean-Sigma goals, the business unit goals (Level II). Panel F will be the place where each team or individual can list their team goals (Level III measurements/goals).

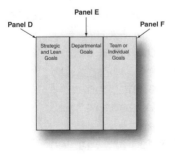

The most important thing to remember about Goal Cards is design follows function. Each healthcare institution should create a design that works for them. And remember, all Goal Cards must be simple and easy to read and use.

How do you do it?

The seven steps to creating Goal Cards are:

1. Articulate a Lean strategy.
2. Identify Lean goals.
3. Create a facility Goal Card.
4. Present the process to the facility.
5. Integrate personal and/or team goals.
6. Post the Goal Card.
7. Continue to monitor and review goals.

1. Articulate a Lean strategy.

Strategic planning has been in existence for many years, but only in the past 10 years or so was the Strategic Plan for an organization deemed a value to share with all employees. Goal Cards focus explicitly on all business processes. This will allow the organization to achieve success. Lean is one of those systems allowing this to occur.

2. Identify Lean goals.

A strategy is useless without direction. This direction is provided by a few solid goals that lend themselves to measurement. Many organizations have had the most success with four types of goals, usually defined as:

• Improved patient satisfaction
• Financial (business) growth
• Process improvement
• Development of organizational learning

Some organizations find it useful to divide process improvement into three goals that include: quality improvement, productivity improvement, and customer/patient satisfaction.

Goals provide an outline for the strategic direction of a facility. Goals must be specific, measurable, and attainable. For example, a goal might be, "To improve patient satisfaction." But everyone wants to do that. So a Lean Goal should give direction to the facility. For example, some Lean goals may appear as follows:

- Reduce patient wait time by 10%
- Reduce the time interval between contacting the office for appointment and seeing the provider by 15%
- Reduce operating room turnover times by 10%
- Reduce supplies by 10%

3. Create a facility Goal Card.

The following should be considered when developing a Goal Card:

- Include the administrator's introduction to all employees
- Write a presentation of Lean Strategy and Goals
- Create a panel for team and/or individual goals
- Print the Goal Card for facility-wide distribution

Now the Goal Card process is ready for implementation.

4. Present the process to the facility.

This can be accomplished through staff meetings. Further communications can occur through the intranet, newsletters, bulletin boards, etc.

5. Integrate personal and/or team goals.

Depending on the size and structure of the facility, this step may involve identifying department or team goals before individuals articulate their personal goals. Whatever the situation, the principles of effective goal setting are the same.

The following guidelines will help keep personal and team goals understandable and useful:

*   Goals should be attainable
*   Goals should be challenging
*   Goals should be meaningful to the individual or team
*   Goals should be based on facility and/or department objectives
*   Goals should be stated simply and clearly

Goals should always include the following:

*   An action verb [to reduce]
*   Measurable output [errors at specific process]
*   Quantity improvement [by 50%]
*   Time frame [by December 22]

6. Post the Goal Card.

The Goal Card should be posted where it can be easily referred to by all staff.

7. Continue to monitor and review goals.

Do not underestimate the power of recognition. A little recognition helps break many barriers within a facility. In addition, people need to feel responsible to peers as well as leaders. Monitoring and visually reporting progress creates a culture of sharing, recognition, and responsibility.

Key Points for the Goal Card in Healthcare

- Create a realistic timeline for developing Goal Cards and implementing them facility-wide.
- Goals Cards should be completed yearly.
- Keep goals realistic and obtainable.
- Management should continually reinforce Goal Cards by giving recognition to the department and individuals when visiting the area.
- Goal Cards should be posted in work areas.
- Goal Cards are a critical element to the Lean and Six Sigma initiatives in the overall facility improvement process.

Case Studies and/or Photos

Emergency Department

The following is an example of a Goal Card for the Emergency Department of a hospital.

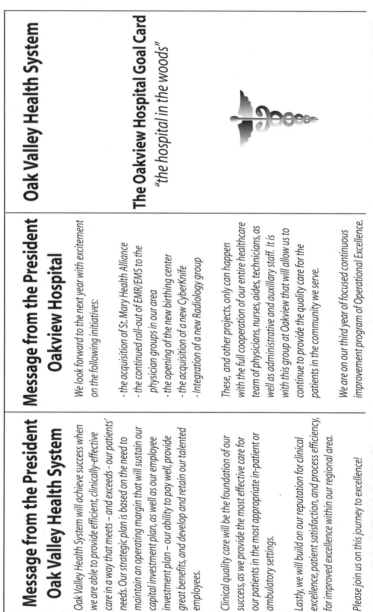

Oak Valley Health System

The Oakview Hospital Goal Card
"the hospital in the woods"

Message from the President Oakview Hospital

We look forward to the next year with excitement on the following initiatives:

- the acquisition of St. Mary Health Alliance
- the continued roll-out of EMR/EMS to the physician groups in our area
- the opening of the new birthing center
- the acquisition of a new CyberKnife
- Integration of a new Radiology group

These, and other projects, only can happen with the full cooperation of our entire healthcare team of physicians, nurses, aides, technicians, as well as administrative and auxillary staff. It is with this group at Oakview that will allow us to continue to provide the quality care for the patients in the community we serve.

We are on our third year of focused continuous improvement program of Operational Excellence.

Message from the President Oak Valley Health System

Oak Valley Health System will achieve success when we are able to provide efficient, clinically-effective care in a way that meets – and exceeds - our patients' needs. Our strategic plan is based on the need to maintain an operating margin that will sustain our capital investment plan, as well as our employee investment plan – our ability to pay well, provide great benefits, and develop and retain our talented employees.

Clinical quality care will be the foundation of our success, as we provide the most effective care for our patients in the most appropriate in-patient or ambulatory settings.

Lastly we will build on our reputation for clinical excellence, patient satisfaction, and process efficiency, for improved excellence within our regional area.

Please join us on this journey to excellence!

We are totally committed to its success. It is through the use of this Goal Card that has assisted us to remain competitive and be in a position of continued growth. Much of this can only occur if the organization is in total alignment.

Your past support in meeting the goals you set forth in the Goal Card is appreciated and I know you will continue that type of support in the coming year.

Sincerely,

John Abrahams, MD
President & CEO, Oakview Hospital

"The Oak Valley Health System is committed to providing personal and high quality state of the art care with compassion and community focus."

Bruce Stubbs, MD
President & CEO, Oak Vally Health System

Janie Rathborne, MSN
Vice President, Patient Services

Dave Hendrix, MBA
Chief Financial Officer

Carrie Millhouse
Vice President, Human Resources

George Thomas, MD
Chief Medical Officer

Vanessa Williams, PhD
Director of Quality Improvement

Oak Valley Health System Strategic Goals

The following goals represent the direction of OVHS. We need to focus our efforts in these areas to provide the infrastructure required to serve our patients and community in the short and long term.

Finance Goals

Operating Margin %:	5.0
Adj Cost per Equiv Admit	7500

Quality

Bundles, % of 100%	100
Mortality Rate, Var from Norm	< -1.0
Falls per 100 Pt Days	< 2.5

Service (Cycle Time)

ED % of Admitted Pts Meeting Target (4.5 hrs)	85
ED LOS for Admit Patients (hrs)	4.5
OR % On-time Case Starts	85
LOS, Med-Surg (Days)	3.5

Oakview Hospital Strategic Goals

In support of the strategic goals of OVHS, we will continue to focus our efforts to improve our goals as they are aligned with the system goals.

Finance Goals

Operating Margin %:	4.0
Adj Cost per Equiv Admit	7500

Quality

Bundles, % of 100%	100
Mortality Rate, Var from Norm	< -1.0
Falls per 100 Pt Days	< 2.5

Service (Cycle Time)

ED % of Admitted Pts Meeting Target (4.5 hrs)	85
OR % On-time Case Starts	85
LOS, Med-Surg (Days)	3.5

ED Goal Card

Value Statement

"The process for admitting a patient has two goals: efficiency in the process and the patient in the right bed the first time. We need to move our admitted patients as quickly as possible to a more clinically appropriate care setting, one that meets the needs of the patients and their families in a less crisis-driven environment."

Team/Department/Individual Goals:

ED Adm Pts LOS <= 4.5 hrs, improve from 6 hrs (25%)

Dispo-to-Admit Cycle Time <= 1.5 hrs, improve by 50%

ED Patient Satisfaction, improve by 50%

Bed/Clothing check >= 95% complete, improve by 50%

Admit Order to Bed Assigned <= 30 min, improve by 50%

Bed Assigned to Pt in Bed <= 30 min, improve by 50%

Satisfaction

Inpt Satisfaction	4.0
ED Satisfaction	4.0
OR Satisfaction	4.0
Physician Satisfaction (quarterly)	4.0
Employee Satisfaction (quarterly)	4.0

Satisfaction

Inpt Satisfaction	4.0
ED Satisfaction	4.0
OR Satisfaction	4.0
Physician Satisfaction (quarterly)	4.0
Employee Satisfaction (quarterly)	4.0

Signatures:

Dave Beck   Judy Carne

Anne Culley   Mary Beth Gasey

Bill Hagan   Tanya Burns

Sue Burns   Mary Martin-Hayes

Margaret Rodriguez   Sarah Schultz

Ben Kingsley, MD   Lisa Helms

Rodney Backus, MD   Mary Potts-Geoffrey, MD

Kathy Janeway

Healthcare Case for Lean

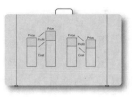

 Why use it?

This will create an understanding for the need to improve healthcare in all its facets. A traditional approach will not work. Healthcare organizations must be run like a successful business, focusing on achieving a positive Return-On-Investment (ROI) by eliminating, or at least minimizing, non value-added activities through the implementation of Lean practices.

Who does it?

The Chief Medical Officer, Chief Executive Officer, Chief Financial Officer (the O's), and/or the Vice President of Quality must present the reasons for adapting Lean as a process improvement system.

How long will it take?

Approximately 1 hour to make the business case.

 What does it do?

It creates the "sense of urgency" within the facility to look at areas that can be improved and do so in a proactive way. It also:

- Communicates a common message to everyone
- Involves the top management immediately
- Creates the foundation for change

How do you do it?

    1. Research how other facilities are using Lean and which competitive factors are a challenge in the local health-care community. Many manufacturing councils are now part-nering with hospitals in sharing how they use Lean. Even though it is manufacturing, the principles can be viewed and adapted.

2. Prepare a presentation to all company employees on what challenges the facility faces. Be as honest as you can with-out comprising competitive information. Many Lean health-care case studies have been documented on the internet. Share a few of these with the staff.

3. Prepare information and data for potential questions that will arise during the meeting. Attempt to predict what the difficult questions will be when the presentation is made. Have as many facts as possible to address proposed ques-tions.

4. Conduct a beta session (selected group of staff for review) to ensure timing, information relevancy, and presentation style are appropriate.

5. Present the information at the staff meeting or at small gath-erings (i.e., town hall meetings, "lunch and learns," etc.).

6. Ensure time is allocated for questions. If at all possible, convey what changes will be forthcoming or what the continued emphasis for the facility will be.

7. Follow-up with conveying the same information in an abbreviated form via the Goal Card, newsletters, bulletin boards, and facility's intranet. Consider posting directions and goals on the facility's web site to communicate the institutions commitment to patient safety, quality, and continuous improvement.

Key Points for the Healthcare Case in Healthcare

- Communicate at all levels of the facility.
- Consider bringing in outside speakers to stress the importance of the change required in healthcare.
- Create regular roundtable sessions to allow staff access to upper management.
- Continue to benchmark (i.e., visit and evaluate) other facilities in the healthcare or manufacturing industry that are practicing Lean or Six Sigma.
- Lean healthcare is a mindset as well as a set of tools.

🍎 Case Studies and/or Photos

Hyperbaric Medicine

One hospital's senior officials planned to construct a new building to house its hyperbaric medicine program. They used Lean principles of waste reduction, 5S, value stream mapping, and physical layout. Thanks to a greater understanding of the Lean tools, the senior officials discovered that the hospital had sufficient space within the existing building. The results were:

1. Savings of $2 million
2. Increased patient satisfaction and safety

Pathology Lab

After a year long effort of 77 empowered workers implementing over 100 process improvements, the surgical pathology cases with in process defects were reduced by 55% to 1 in 8 cases and timeliness of routine biopsy reports completed within one day improved by 19%. The changes made here were due largely to:

- Leadership providing the vision, structure, resources and managerial expectation to change to a culture of an empowered, enabled workforce
- Creating measurement tools enabling workers to blamelessly expose and capture in real-time in-process defects and waste
- Establishing an expectation of routine communication between work areas (cells)
- Requiring a scientific data-based approach for testing and accepting changes
- Allowing all staff to continuously learn and improve by being empowered to identify the numerous sources of waste and design effective improvements in pursuit of a 'zero defect' performance goal

Interruptions and Random Arrivals

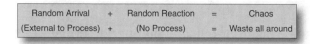

Random Arrival	+	Random Reaction	=	Chaos
(External to Process)	+	(No Process)	=	Waste all around

Why use it?

This will allow you to diligently acknowledge when non-essential work interruptions occur and the reason.

Who does it?

All staff will document interruptions for up to 1 month.

How long does it take?

It takes only seconds per day to accomplish this task.

What does it do?

Collecting the information regarding an interruption during the course of day brings attention to the actual value-added time. Every time there is an interruption, some type of waste is caused. An interruption is defined as a disruption to someone that is working on a process or task (or an unscheduled event).

The documentation of these interruptions will accomplish the following:

- Create awareness of organizational time
- Improve productivity as staff may be reluctant to interrupt someone knowing it will be documented
- Identify how often interruptions occur, from both internal and external sources

How do you do it?

1. Communicate to the team that interruptions need to be documented.

Explain the concept of Random Arrival. Interruptions are often referred to as "Random Arrivals" because you never know when one will occur. This will initiate or cause a "Random Reaction" from the staff once they have been interrupted.

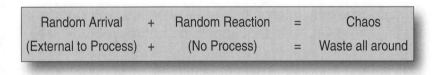

| Random Arrival | + | Random Reaction | = | Chaos |
| (External to Process) | + | (No Process) | = | Waste all around |

2. Create an Interruption and Random Arrival Log.

The Interruption and Random Arrival Log will identify how much time is lost during the day. It will also identify the following:

- How often interruptions stop work
- How much time is consumed or "lost" when the interruption occurs
- The cause of the interruption

Interruption and Random Arrival Log					
Name _____ Month _____					
Department _____ Job Title or Function _____					
No.	Date	Start Time	End Time	Name	Discussion Topic
1					
2					
3					

3. Collect Interruption Log data for 1 month.

This will provide the snapshot required to further focus the team. The Interruption Log then could be used every six months to continually bring awareness to the importance of organizational time.

4. Analyze the data collected.

This can be accomplished by the Lean project team. If someone is consistently interrupting other workers with non value-added information, then that should be addressed privately.

5. Utilize Lean tools to reduce, eliminate, or control the interruptions.

If someone constantly is being interrupted because he or she is the only person that can assist the process due to his or her expertise, then standard work and cross-training is required.

There is no winner when interruptions occur. Any task or process can be affected by random arrival. It is unavoidable. Lean must include a process to assist in identifying, containing, and scheduling the facility-needed interruptions within a controlled environment. This creates less frequent interruptions. If interruptions are part of the required service, then standards need to be created and followed to address them.

Key Points for Interruptions and Random Arrivals in Healthcare

- Communicate, communicate, and communicate to the staff the importance of organizational time.
- Ensure everyone understands that interruptions (i.e., random arrivals) cause waste.
- Utilize the Interruption Log for everyone, including the manager/supervisor. If he or she is constantly interrupting a staff member, this needs to be documented.
- Keep the larger picture of Lean Healthcare in mind. The Interruption Log is only temporary.
- Most likely 80% of the interruptions will be documented. Accept that number and work with it.

Just-In-Time (JIT)

Supplier   Customer

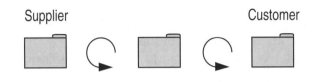

 Why use it?

JIT establishes a system of supplying service to the internal or external customer, patient, or healthcare provider at precisely the right time, in the correct amounts, and without error.

Note: external or internal customers may be other healthcare providers or facilities, satellite offices, or labs.

Who does it?

The Lean project team will determine the need for JIT. Additional Lean tools will be required to implement this concept. Eventually, everyone in the value stream will contribute to JIT.

How long does it take?

This is a long term cognitive and cultural change. However, to get started, it may take anywhere from a few weeks to months to bring awareness to the concept.

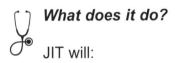 **What does it do?**

JIT will:

- Typically utilize new physical layouts (See Physical Layout)
- Allow work to flow between processes with minimal or no wait time

- Improve departmental, facility, and/or staff productivity by reducing transport and motion wastes (See Waste)
- Improve quality at the source of information, service, or care by identifying problems earlier

How do you do it?

1. Takt time is to be used in conjunction with continuous flow tools. (See Takt Time)

2. Implement continuous flow tools to establish communication that will balance cycle times to allow work to flow or provide a service at a steady pace.

3. Utilize kanbans as part of the Pull System and create visuals for easier understanding. (See Pull Systems)

4. Monitor continuous flow tools and proceed to JIT.

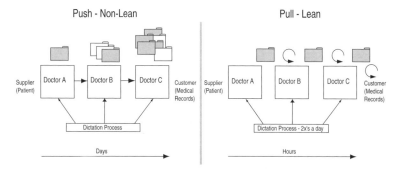

In a clinic, doctors may delay their chart dictation for a day due to an increase in the number of patients being seen, which may then accumulate for up to 3 days. A Lean approach would have them schedule time twice a day to dictate medical records for that day. This will also level the work for medical records, in that they would be receiving dictation in smaller amounts with increased frequency. This would allow the work to flow at a more steady pace.

Key Points for JIT in Healthcare

- This principle applies to both internal and external customers (i.e., patients, facilities, departments, healthcare providers, etc.).
- JIT is the overriding theme for Lean healthcare.
- JIT is the big picture and will not be attained overnight.
- JIT will assist in identifying problems early on.
- JIT will allow for a drastic reduction in wait times.
- Continue to make minor adjustments to the system by gathering improvement ideas from the staff.

Kaizen Events

 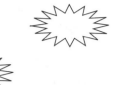

 ## *Why use it?*

Kaizen Events enable you to learn and implement continuous improvement practices (i.e., Lean tools) by a
group of individuals to a targeted area within a specified time period.

Who does it?

The Lean project team will be responsible for planning and
implementing the Lean tools. All employees should be doing
their own kaizen daily.

How long does it take?

This is a long term cognitive and cultural change. A Kaizen
Event may last 1 - 2 days, or may be broken up into manageable action items during a period of time.

What does it do?

Kaizen - "Kai" means to "take apart" and "zen" means to
"make good." Kaizen is synonymous with continuous
improvement.

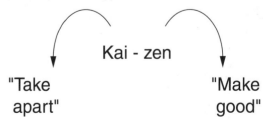

Kai - zen

"Take   "Make
apart"   good"

Kaizen Events will accomplish the following:

- Quickly implement Lean tools to eliminate waste and non value-added work
- Train staff in Lean tools and applications
- Improve work flow
- Improve productivity
- Reduce stress

How do you do it?

There are three phases to conducting a Kaizen Event:

1. Planning Phase
2. Kaizen Workshop Phase
3. Follow-Up Phase

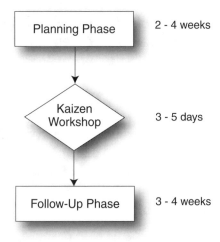

1. Planning Phase

a. Create a current and future state value stream or process map. Use this road map to identify problems or areas in which waste can be eliminated. (See Value Stream Mapping)

b. Assemble the core Kaizen team. This should be made up of a multi-disciplinary group of workers.

c. Complete a Team Charter with the Kaizen team. Ensure a project champion has been identified. (See Reporting and Communications)

d. Obtain approval for the Team Charter from the champion. A project champion is a management position that has the authority to commit facility resources. Solicit input and update the Charter as necessary.

e. Communicate to staff who will be affected by the event well before it begins. Make sure everyone understands how this kaizen activity will affect them and what may be expected from them. Post the Team Charter.

f. Create a Kaizen Milestone Worksheet (also referred to as a Project Checklist) to detail the improvement activities.

Kaizen Milestone Worksheet

Value Stream ___Supply Room - 7th Floor___ Date _6/22/05_ Page _1_ of _2_

Department _Nursing_____

Specific Event	Person	Date Assigned	Date Completed
5S - Sort out supplies in cabinets	D.T.	6/22	6/29
Create initial supply survey form	S.M.	6/22	

2. Kaizen Workshop Phase

g. Train the team in Lean concepts.

h. Begin the workshop by applying 5S.

i. Observe the area that is to be improved and see how it currently works. Gather accurate data on cycle times. (See Cycle Time)

j. Break the team into smaller groups to brainstorm for ways to improve the area(s) that are part of the event.

k. Implement improvements from the brainstorming session(s). Create specific tasks. List all activities that require completion after the event on the Kaizen Milestone Worksheet.

3. Follow-Up Phase

l. Report results obtained to the champion.

m. Continue to implement ideas from the Kaizen Milestone Worksheet. Once processes have been improved, create standards. (See Standard Work)

n. Submit regular Status Reports to the champion. This communicates the status of the project.

o. Submit a final report when the Kaizen Event is completed.

Key Points for Kaizen Events in Healthcare

- A proper Kaizen Event will have all three phases.
- The Planning Phase and Follow-Up Phase are just as important as the Workshop Phase.
- Kaizen Events can be focused on one area or process, or on multiple areas.
- Kaizen Events can be successful only if management (champion) is in support and there is cooperation from the staff.
- Keep Kaizen Events manageable with focused projects. Expand as you experience success.
- Always keep 5S as an initial part of any Kaizen Event. Even if you plan to install an entire software program as a Kaizen Event, consider applying 5S principles to everyone's Desktop PC file system - first.

🍎 Case Studies and/or Photos

Outcomes Management

One hospital hired a Vice President of Outcomes Management to oversee Lean projects. Considerable staff training was done to ensure top management understood why the Lean system needed to be utilized. It was decided that 2 Kaizen Events (each 3 days in length) would be conducted each month. Each Kaizen Event consisted of the following:

Day 1 am - Lean Tools Definitions and Case Studies
Day 1 pm - Obstacles to Change and Creation of Current State Value Stream or Process Map
Day 2 am - Continuation of Value Stream Mapping and time observations
Day 2 pm - Selected Lean tools were applied to appropriate areas for testing and feasibility
Day 3 am - Future State Value Stream Maps were created
Day 3 pm - 15 minute presentations to the Chief Medical Officer, Chief Financial Officer, Chief Executive Officer, etc. on the Lean project. Determination of resources and continuation of project(s) decided.

This resulted in the following outcomes:

1. Increased profitability by 12% over the previous non-Lean year
2. Improved nurse satisfaction and staff satisfaction
3. $500,000 cost savings realized
4. Staff job interest increased by additional staff volunteering to be part of Kaizen Events

Kanbans for Supplies

Supply Re-order Kanban Card
Item Name: _____
Maximum Quanity: _____
Minimum Quantity: _____
Re-order Quantity: _____ (Max - Min)
Vendor Name: _____ Catalog Page No: ____
Place this card in the Kanban Envelope

Why use it?

Kanbans create a Pull System for supplies that reduces waste of motion and transport. This will also reduce inventory.

Who does it?

The Lean project team made up of representatives from the department or area served by the supplies.

How long does it take?

It will take only a few hours for meetings and initial setup.

What does it do?

A kanban is a means of communicating via a signal (i.e., card, tag, folder, email, etc.) to an upstream process precisely what is required at the time it is required. The Kanbans for Supplies will ensure the dollars allocated for supplies will be at the minimum required. The Kanban System is used to create a "pull" of material, in this case an supply item, from a upstream process to a downstream process.

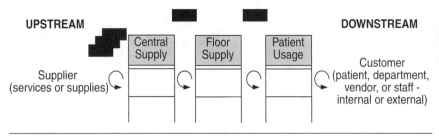

The system utilizes a Lean tool known as a Kanban to ensure equipment, material, service, or supply will be available when required, in the correct quantity.

How do you do it?

There are eight steps to creating and implementing the Kanban System for Supplies. They are:

1. Conduct the supply survey.
2. Establish minimum/maximum levels.
3. Create the Supply Order Form.
4. Create the Kanban cards.
5. Create standard work. (See Standard Work)
6. Conduct the training.
7. Implement the Kanban System.
8. Maintain the standards.

1. Conduct the supply survey.

The team will need to create a standard list of supplies from which to draw upon. Following is a sample Supply Survey Form.

Supply Survey Form		
Please indicate from the list below the frequency of the items you will most likely use within a specific time period. (i.e., shift, day, week, or month). This data will be used to assist the Lean project team to establish the quantity of supplies to assure the item is there when you need it. Also, any items not listed, please add to the bottom of the form.		
Item Description	**Quantity Used/Time Period**	**Comments**
Exam Gloves #7 (box)	0.5 box/shift (50 gloves)/shift	
Paper Drapes (50/box)	10/shift	
General Use Syringes - 3ml	50/shift	

2. Establish minimum/maximum levels.

Once the list and special requests have been collected, gain a consensus on usage and establish minimum/maximum levels. Include the following:

- Type of standard supply (there are numerous glove sizes, agree on a certain quantity for each size)
- Weekly or monthly usage for the items
- Establish a minimum quantity to have on hand
- Establish a maximum quantity to have on hand

3. Create the Supply Order Form.

This form will list all the supplies represented by information obtained from the Supply Survey Form. Once the team has established the type of supplies, minimum and maximum levels need to be determined. The minimum quantity to have on hand is the quantity of items expected to be used during the time it takes to re-supply that item (plus some X factor or buffer). The maximum quantity to have on hand will be the minimum quantity plus the number of items that would be used during the supply or replenishment time.

Supply Order Form

Please fax this form to Central Supply, ext. 2234 by 1700 each day. The supplies will be delivered by 0800 the next day.

Delivery Location: _Pediatrics - Nurse Station_   Account Number: _PD5602_

No.	Item Description	Item #	Quantity Ordered Max - Min	Unit Price
1	Exam Gloves #7 (box)	GLEM70	2	$7.95
2	Paper Drapes (50/box)	DR33656	4	$17.68
3	General Use Syringes - 3ml	SP86A	100	$0.16
4				

Example:
>Item: size 7 latex gloves, 20 used per shift, (3 shifts)
>Total usage of size 7 latex gloves for a day: averages 60 (20 per shift x 3 shifts)
>Order quantity: Size 7 latex gloves are purchased in boxes of 100. The additional 40 per box could be considered the built in X factor or buffer per day. The buffer of 40 gloves would need to be reviewed monthly and adjustments to the order would need to be done to ensure of not overstocking the size 7 latex gloves.
>Re-order time from central supply: 2 days

Minimum Required: 1 box (100 gloves)
Maximum Number: 3 boxes (300 gloves)
Re-order time from Central Supply: 2 days

4. Create the Kanban cards.

There should be one Kanban card identified as the Supply Re-order Kanban for each supply item. It should be laminated and color-coded differentiating more than one supply ordering location (i.e., Baxter, Central Supply, Staples, etc.). Kanban cards should be affixed to the minimum re-order quantity item. For example, attach the Kanban card to the last box of gloves on the shelf.

The card should be an appropriate size to visually convey all the pertinent information such as:

>Item Name
>Maximum Quantity on Hand
>Minimum Quantity on Hand
>Re-order Quantity (Maximum - Minimum)
>Vendor Name
>Catalog Page Number
>Instructions as to what to do with the Kanban card

The following is an example of a Kanban card:

Supply Re-order Kanban Card	
Item Name: Size #7 latex gloves	
Maximum Quantity: 3 boxes - (100 pair/box)	
Minimum Quantity: 1 box - (100 pair/box)	
Re-order Quantity: 2 boxes **(Max - Min)**	
Vendor Name: Central Supply **Catalog Pg. No:** N/A	
Place this card in the Kanban Envelope	

Note: Ensure a Special Order Kanban Card is created to be filled in by the staff for those special order items (e.g., latex-free band-aids). Typically there will not be a minimum/maximum number. Monitor Special Order Kanbans to determine if they should be included on the Supply Order Form.

5. Create standard work.

Once the system has been designed and the process for re-ordering determined, create a Standard Work Chart. This should be posted at the supply cabinet and used to train the staff. (See Standard Work)

6. Conduct the training.

The training for the department should be done prior to implementation to ensure integrity of the system. The training should include the following:

- A brief explanation of the purpose of Kanbans
- Explanation of how the minimum/maximum levels were established and convey appreciation of everyone's input when the Supply Survey was conducted
- Explanation of how the system will work (distribute process flowcharts)

- Explanation of the two types of kanbans: Supply Re-order and Special Order Kanban
- A demonstration at the supply cabinet on the location and placement of the Kanbans. Also, a demonstration of where the Kanbans are to be placed once the item category has reached its minimum inventory level and re-ordering is required.
- Acknowledgement of the key individuals within the team that contributed to this system

Note: Understand that this is a work-in-progress trial and improvement ideas from all staff will be welcomed.

7. Implement the Kanban System.

Training and implementation should occur simultaneously. Once the training has been completed, the Kanban for Supplies will be ready for usage.

8. Maintain the standards.

After a month or two of usage, review the appropriate budget supply line item. Determine the cost savings and congratulate the team. Convey success to management. Continue to take suggestions on how the process can be improved.

Include 5S as part of the process.

The benefits of Kanbanning supplies are:

- Ensures minimum inventory
- Creates staff awareness of the cost of supplies
- Easy tool to implement and train
- Encourages teamwork
- Minimizes transactions on ordering supplies
- Reduces stress
- Reduces excess inventory waste

Key Points for Kanbans for Supplies in Healthcare

- Ensure you have a process in place for Special Order Kanbans.
- Consider rotating responsibility for maintaining the system on a monthly or quarterly basis, or other time deemed appropriate for your work area. This will allow more people to be involved in the process and contribute improvement ideas.
- Establish a time to review minimum/maximum levels of supplies and adjust as necessary.
- If appropriate, work with local vendors to keep on-site inventory supply levels at a minimum.
- Use this as a learning tool. Continue to understand and implement JIT techniques and kanbans for work documents, charts, lab requests, etc.

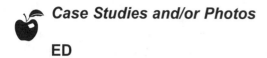

Case Studies and/or Photos

ED

The ED staff complained that they were always running out of items, even though there was someone assigned every day (on the midnight shift) to count and replace inventory. In some cases, small items such as pulse oximeters, were taken with the patients to the inpatient units. In other cases, the last item in stock would be taken, and the next person who needed it would be out of luck. The midnight shift stated that they had a hard time counting everything because there were so many places in the ED where items might be stored. The day shift said they had to stock extra supplies around the ED to make sure they would not run out. It seemed to be a vicious cycle.

The ED Manager decided to spend a week to conduct a supply survey. Each team member was asked to document the amount of each item used, and whether any item was not available when needed.

After looking at the data, a small "Kanban" team determined standards for what (non-medication) items should be stocked in each ED room, and what should be kept in the Clean Utility Room or other appropriate areas. They discussed the ideas and received additional input from the staff at the weekly staff meeting. The team emphasized that an X factor (or buffer) would be kept so that the staff would not run out. Special attention was paid to any items that had expiration dates, to ensure that a surplus would not result in the wasting of these items.

The Kanban team posted minimum and maximum amounts for each item to be stored and then labeled all the areas in the ED rooms where small amounts of material were to be kept on hand. They also created Re-Order and Special-Order Kanban cards for the storage areas and then put together a supply order form with all of those items listed, plus leaving space for special items to be added. The Kanban standard work was posted in the Clean Utility Room. These activities took about three weeks.

Training was done at a weekly staff meeting and the Kanban process was started that day. The Kanban cards were placed at the minimum inventory level (placed between items or taped to the next item), and when visible, would be placed in a special In Box for the midnight shift person designated to do the ordering. The order form would be completed and processed appropriately, i.e., sent via interdepartmental mail or faxed to the vendor before the end of the shift. The order forms were kept in a designated file folder in the Clean Utility Room for easy reference.

When supplies were received, they were processed as usual with the invoices and receivers being signed and sent to the appropriate department. The concept of FIFO was used to make sure that the oldest items would be used first. The Kanban cards were replaced (or attached) at the point of minimum inventory.

The ED staff agreed to review the process on a monthly basis to ensure that it was working as designed. At first the team found a few "hiccups" as some Kanban cards were not placed in the In Box, but after a review of the new process at the weekly meeting, the process was smoothed out. The Kanban team was later recognized at a monthly leadership meeting.

The results after 3 months were:

1. Reduction in $1,256.00 per month in purchased supplies, totalling $3,768.00.
2. Decrease in expired medications, from 1.8% to less than 1% per month, equating to a cost savings of $476.00 per month, totaling $1,428.00.

Leveling

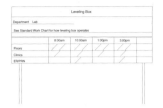

Why use it?

Leveling balances the volume and variety of work among the staff during a period of time - typically a day. It is also known as Heijunka.

Who does it?

A multi-disciplinary team is responsible for this task.

How long does it take?

Once continuous flow has been achieved to the fullest possible extent, this system will tie all the work and processes together. Typically, smaller facilities with less than 200 employees can reach this point in less than a year. Larger facilities may take 1 – 2 years.

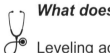

What does it do?

Leveling accomplishes the following:

- Balances work loads and duties of staff where appropriate, considering certifications, licensing, and training
- Provides a visual system for identifying if work is behind schedule
- Reduces wait times
- Assists to achieve continuous work flow

How do you do it?

1. Calculate takt time. (See Takt Time)

Takt time = <u>Available daily work time</u> = <u>Time</u>
Total daily volume required   Volume

2. Determine pitch for each value stream.

Pitch is a multiple of takt time that will allow you to create and maintain a consistent and practical work flow throughout the value stream or area. To calculate pitch, multiply the takt time by the number of work units to flow through the value stream.

Pitch = takt time x practical number of work flow units (or documents)

Example 1:
Takt time: 5 minutes for a blood draw
Optimal number of blood draws to be moved throughout the value stream: 24

Pitch = 5 minutes (takt time) x 24 blood draws (practical number of work flow units) = 120 minute (or 2 hour) pitch

This means every 2 hours the group of 24 blood draws will be moved within the value stream (for all non-stat requests).

Example 2:
Often during rounds the healthcare provider will take all the charts of the patients, complete the rounds, and write orders. This leaves all these charts to be processed at once. Using the concept of pitch, the healthcare provider would complete a subset of that group (maybe 3 of the 12 patient charts) and transport those to the unit manager or coordinator to be processed, and then continue seeing 3 more patients. This will reduce the stress of the unit manager or coordinator and reduce any potential for error.

3. Create work sequence.

Actual times must be established to move the work at the pitch increments. From example 1, the pitch increment would be 2 hours.

0800   0900   1000   1100   1200   etc.

4. Create a Leveling Sequence Table.

A Leveling Sequence Table is a matrix showing the times for each value stream process and the correct quantity of work to be processed. This table shows the whole story of work processes at a glance and should be posted. This should be recalculated as requirements change.

Leveling Sequence Table (routine)										
Customers (i.e., value streams)	Pitch (minutes)	Daily Pick-Up Times with Number of Units (Day Shift)								
		0800	0900	1000	1100	1200	1300	1400	1500	1600
Walk-Ins	240					12				12
Pediatrics	120			4		4		4		4
Outpatient Clinics	60				16				16	
Hospital Floors	120		12		12		12		12	

5. Create a leveling box.

A leveling box is a physical device - like a mailbox - that will hold a certain quantity of work that must be processed (or picked up to be processed). It should be clearly identified as such with the Work Sequence Table posted as a visual aid.

6. Put the leveling box into operation.

This will require a runner or someone responsible for picking up and delivering what is in the leveling box (i.e., work units) to the specified area(s) of the value stream.

Key Points for Leveling in Healthcare

- Pitch increments for leveling are recommended to be at least two hours. Smaller increments of time may create more transport and motion waste than is necessary.
- The leveling device should be placed in a common area. It is recommended that one value stream be created and loaded into the device, and then additional ones be added once it is working efficiently. For example, in the Emergency Room, the leveling box may have slots for (1) labs to be picked up, (2) X-rays to be processed, and (3) physician orders to be processed.
- Each slot within the leveling box should be labeled with the pitch times.
- The Work Sequence Table and Standard Work Chart should be posted at the leveling device location.

Case Studies and/or Photos

Trauma Center

A large trauma center hospital experienced a chronic problem with a lack of beds on its surgical step down unit, especially on Wednesdays and Thursdays. The elective surgery schedule had a problem with flow due to add-ons of 15 to 20 patients per day and a 20% cancellation rate.

A review of the surgery schedule revealed that Vascular Services performed their surgeries in batches, four cases one day and none the next. Administration worked with Vascular Services to limit the number of patients going to the step down unit each day to two. The vascular surgeons were offered more surgery time on Mondays and Fridays in exchange. This change resulted in smoother case flow and 50% fewer nursing hours per patient per day in the step down unit. The results were:

1. Smoother patient flow
2. Decrease in nursing hours in the step down unit
3. Improved patient satisfaction
4. Reduced the cancellation rate by 50%, to less than 10%

Lab

The laboratory serviced a number of local nursing homes as well as outpatient clinics. Couriers were sent out throughout the day and evening to pick up specimens as calls were received. The laboratory looked at their call frequency to see if they could use a leveling or pitch strategy to better service the demands that were occurring throughout the day and make more efficient use of the courier service.

Takt Times for Lab Pick-ups				
Value Stream	Daily Time Available (day + afternoon shifts)	Daily Volume of Work	Time / Volume	Takt Time (minutes)
Nursing Homes	960	17 specimens from 12 nursing homes	960 / 17	56
Outpatient Clinics	960	60 specimens from 6 outpatient clinics	960 / 60	16

Pitch Time for Lab Pick-ups			
Value Stream	Takt Time (minutes)	Optimal Number of Work Units to Flow	Takt Time X Optimal Number of Work Units to Flow
Nursing Homes	56	4	224
Outpatient Clinics	16	15	240

The lab team decided that if they picked up specimens every 4 hours (240 minutes) they would usually have 3 - 5 specimens to pick up from the nursing homes, as well as 25 - 30 from the outpatient clinics, which made a courier run worthwhile. The first pick-up would be done with the morning blood specimen collection, at 0700 - 0800, so the rest of the routine courier pick-ups could be spaced 4 hours apart, 1100, 1500, 1900, and 2300. (The latter two times would not be scheduled for the outpatient clinics.)

The leveling sequence table looked like this:

Heiunka Box (or Leveling Visual)						
Value Stream	Pitch Time (minutes)	Daily Pick-up Times with Number of Units (Days + Afternoons)				
		0700	1100	1500	1900	2300
Nursing Homes	224 (approx. 4 hours)	3-5	3-5	3-5	3-5	3-5
Outpatient Clinics	240 (4 hours)		25-30	25-30		

The courier runs were minimized, and the nursing homes and clinics no longer had to call for each specimen, since the pickup runs were made regularly. They subsequently stan-dardized the daily pick-up times to be 1100 and 1500. This reduced the number of those additional trips by 10 per month, at an average cost of $154.00 per trip, for a cost savings of $1540.00 per month.

Measurement Techniques

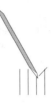

 Why use it?

This tool accurately and efficiently collects information relative to patient or healthcare provider demand. This will allow the team and the manager to allocate the appropriate staff and resources to ensure patient and healthcare provider needs are met.

Who does it?

Staff will need to collect relevant data.

How long will it take?

It will take only a few minutes per day. If urgency is an issue, then a minimum three month historical trend can be utilized. This may take 2 - 3 hours to collect and summarize.

What does it do?

Data will be required to calculate takt time. This can be collected by providing the worker with the Data Capture Form to identify the work they are currently doing. The team should create a standard form that lists the various common duties that are being performed. Then the worker only needs to check-off when the duty is performed. (See Takt Time)

Good data collection techniques provide the following:

- A good baseline upon which to utilize Lean tools and concepts
- An awareness of the actual work being done and by whom it is being done by
- Known duties that are being done, as well as those "other" duties that occupy people's time

 ### How do you do it?

The following steps can be used to accurately collect information for value stream projects.

1. Brainstorm with the team to generate a list of common duties in the department or what has been determined to be the value stream (i.e., other departments, etc.). (See Value Stream Mapping)

2. Create a Data Capture Form that will list the duties from Step 1. Ensure the form has additional space to document duties not listed.

Everyone is a customer to someone else. The patient is the ultimate customer. Think of a river - it flows downstream from an upstream source to a lake, ocean, or sea. All services flow downstream to where the patient (or customer) is. The supplier of service can be the doctor, lab, or anyone who renders service to the patient. For example, a pharmacy can be the upstream process (e.g., supplier) to the downstream process (e.g., customer) in dispersing medications. The downstream customer in this case can be the nurse that is dispersing the medications or the patient that receives the meds.

3. Utilize the form for a given period of time to ensure you are aware of all the activities and processes related to the value stream.

4. Consolidate the report.

5. Identify common duties that serve multiple value streams. For example, the lab may service different departments such as the Emergency Rooms, operating rooms, floors, etc. Each may have varying requests.

6. Calculate takt time. (See Takt Time)

7. Create a plan to ensure takt time is met using appropriate Lean tools.

8. Create a "help" tool. For example, if you are performing multiple tasks in the lab and have a specific time limit for completion, a help tool, such as a "Do Not Disturb" sign, may be useful as a visual aid in communicating that a customer demand must be met.

Takt time will eventually become a common word within healthcare. Takt time should be made visible to staff. This can be accomplished by creating a placard with the takt time displayed at the point of use.

The benefits of good measurement techniques are:

- Creates awareness of the importance of takt time
- Compliments the efforts of Lean activities
- Improves productivity by paying constant attention to what needs to be completed to meet a patient or healthcare provider request

Distribution Report

Another option would be to utilize historical data on patient (or customer) demand if it is available. This should include at least 3 months worth of data. After the raw data for the processes within the value stream has been collected, a Distribution Report should be created.

Distribution/Volume Report

Department Oakview Hospital   **Data Collection Dates** March 1 - 31

Type of Data Collection
- ✓ Historical (database retrieval)
- Direct Observation (real time)
- Voice of the Customer (survey)

Department (reasons why pts come to the hospital	Pts/month	Registration	OP Scheduling	Transport	Housekeeping	Medical Records
IP visit/surgery	457	X		X	X	X
OP Surgery	140	X	X	X	X	X
OP Laboratory	230	X				X
OP Radiology	160	X	X		X	X
Clinic visit	178	X	X		X	X
ED visit	**2950**	**X**		**X**	**X**	**X**
Outpt Pharmacy visit	124					X
OP Phys/Occ Therapy	85	X	X		X	X
Community classes	425				X	X
Pt visitors - # of visits	1156					

Key Points for Measurement Techniques in Healthcare

- Do not collect the micro details of the duties at this stage. Other Lean tools will be used for that.
- Focus on the duties the staff are doing, ensure they feel comfortable being honest in capturing the data.
- Be supportive.
- Managers and supervisors must set the example. Even though their duties are different, managers and supervisors should be included in as much of the data collection as possible.

Paper File System

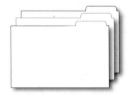

Why use it?

This system ensures paperwork is organized and processed correctly. This is an integral part of the facility paper system. It can assist work flow in finance, billing, administration, and patient scheduling. Almost every outpatient clinical area has a front office area - cardiac cath, radiology, endoscopy, laboratory, sleep lab, etc., that can benefit from using all or parts of what is contained in this section.

Who does it?

The Lean project team will work to create the file system with input from all staff. Everyone will eventually be required to follow the new paper file system standards.

How long will it take?

This will require regular, ongoing meetings for designing, implementing, and maintaining the paper file system.

What does it do?

The paper file system will consist of creating and maintaining three types of folders: the system folder, the process folder, and the reference folder. Each of these folders will contain the actual process work or information required to run the system. Later in this section each of these folders will be addressed in detail.

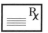

How do you do it?

There is a three step procedure for this section. The steps are:

1. Create the system folder.
2. Create the process folder (or Kanban) and reference folder.
3. Establish a holding point.

Note: This is the most time consuming section in *The New Lean Healthcare Pocket Guide XL*. Note: As organizations continue the migration to a paperless system, consider the concepts in this chapter to be applied to what currently is paper-based. These tools and concepts can also be applied to your electronic files and folders.

1. Create the system folder.

The system folder will be the "headquarters" of all pertinent information about the processes or value streams. It is the organized listing (i.e., processes) of the work for the entire Lean system. The system folder will:

- Centralize all process information
- Create a visual aid for document control (having a list of all processes in a document within a system folder)
- Support continuous improvement
- Allow for process knowledge to be further owned and understood by the facility and staff

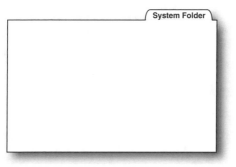

A. Inside of system folder

Inside of the system folder will be the "brains" of the entire Lean Office. It will contain the Process Master Document, Process Review Schedule, and the Training Matrix. Other documents may be included to support the overall concept of the system folder.

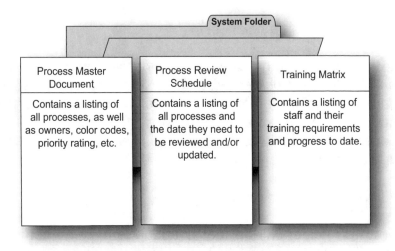

Process Master Document	Process Review Schedule	Training Matrix
Contains a listing of all processes, as well as owners, color codes, priority rating, etc.	Contains a listing of all processes and the date they need to be reviewed and/or updated.	Contains a listing of staff and their training requirements and progress to date.

B. Outside of system folder

The outside of the system folder will have the folder priority rating displayed and the status of the folder. The folder priority rating is a color-coded visual aid representing each type of process. A color will be assigned to Critical 1, 2, 3 (multiple colors may be assigned), Non-Critical, and Reference processes.

Critical is defined as those administrative processes that directly impact the financial status of the facility (e.g., patient wait time, Operating Room turn-around time, patient or staff satisfaction).

Non-critical is defined as those processes that are necessary, but do not have an immediate financial impact on the facility (e.g., performance appraisals, interviews, etc.).

Reference information is defined as information required on an as-needed basis (e.g., Standards of Service, Standard Operating Procedures, Policy Manuals, Supply Ordering Catalogs, Audit Information, etc.).

A legend representing the status of the process folder should be displayed on the outside of the folder as a visual aid. A process folder can be in an active or passive state.

An **active state folder** would contain work that needs to be completed and should reside in a horizontal position.

Active State

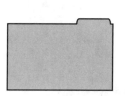

An **passive state folder** would contain work that has already been completed and should reside in a vertical position.

Passive State

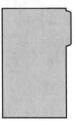

The active or passive state visual cue will accomplish the following:

- Standard communications as to what work is being performed and what is not
- Identification to the manager/supervisor/coach when work is piling up
- Identification of when work has been completed

The system folder should always remain in the active state. The process folder will start out in the active state. It will be moved to a passive state once the work (customer demand) is completed.

The active or passive state should be graphically displayed on the outside of the folder.

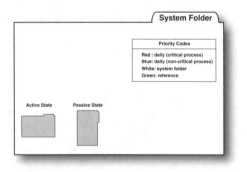

C. Process Master Document

Just as with the Supply Order Form (listing all the various supplies required in the section Kanbans for Supplies), the various processes need to be identified before the process folder for each is created. This will be accomplished by the creation of the Process Master Document. The Process Master Document contains a listing of all the processes required to meet a customer demand.

The Process Master Document electronic version should be maintained and secured by the departmental manager. The hardcopy will be contained in the System Folder.

The six parts to the Process Master Document are:

1. Prioritization and classification of processes
2. Identification of process owners (process owners are those individuals who can perform that process at an expertise level and will maintain the standard in practice and in writing)
3. Determination of color codes (color codes are a visual aid to communicate the priority level of a process)
4. Creation of process flowcharts (See Value Stream Mapping)
5. Validation of the processes (verification the process is currently being run the best way)
6. Train staff of the process(es)

Remember, these are guidelines and the team should discuss what will work best given the requirements of the facility.

2. Create the process folder (or kanban) and reference folder.

Using all process names collected from Step 1, a separate folder for each process will be created. (These will be referred to as process folders, work kanbans, or simply kanbans.)

There are three parts to the process folder:

1. The actual work
2. Process flowchart of standard work (See Standard Work)
3. Volume capture, which is to identify the cycle time that a process requires (See the Value-Added Time Reporting Log later in this section.)

A process folder is located at point-of-use. It is the working document required to ensure the process steps are done in a consistent manner, to the standards set forth by the owner of that process (which follows facility policy). The information contained in the folder will contribute dramatically to reducing work variation through following a standard. This improves work quality.

A process folder is the "keeper" of all working knowledge required to complete that process. It will also contain the actual work required by the customer (i.e., another department, healthcare provider, vendor, etc.). Each process listed in the Process Master Document must have its own process folder.

A process folder will:

• Detail all tasks necessary to complete the process
• Serve as a visual tool to ensure consistent work is accomplished
• Support continuous improvement
• Allow process knowledge to be further owned and understood by the facility

A. Inside of process folder

The process folder will contain the Value-Added Time Reporting Log, Process Flowchart, and the work that must be completed. Remember, the folder is a "Kanban." It is a signal to do work. Later is this chapter you will determine how much work should be placed in each folder.

The Process Flowchart should be placed as the first document within the process folder. It is recommended the flowchart reside in a clear document sleeve for ease of retrieval so improvement ideas can be documented.

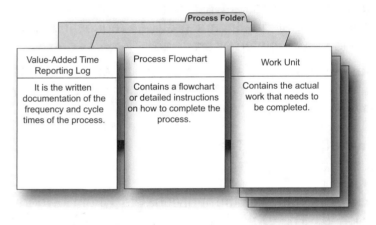

B. Outside of process folder

The outside of the process folder will be labeled in two locations: a label placed on the front of the folder and the other on the tab identifying the process.

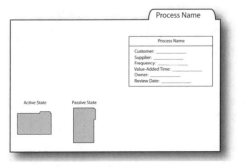

The labeling will be used as a visual aid for quick retrieval of the folder. It will also contribute towards eliminating the waste of waiting.

The following information should be standard on every folder:

Process Name: The name of the process as it is listed on the Process Master Document.

Supplier: The most upstream process supplying work requirements for the department or value stream.

Customer: The most downstream name of the department, process, or other healthcare provider requesting work or a service to be completed or provided.

Frequency: The average number of times the process will need to be completed each day, week, or month. This will be preliminary and subject to change.

Value-Added Time: The total cycle time to complete the process.

Owner: The name of the individual to whom ownership is established. The owner is an individual who can perform that process at an expertise level and will maintain the standard in practice and in writing.

Review Date: The date the process must be reviewed for improvements and/or revisions.

This information should be affixed to each folder. Initially, create a few process folders and then gradually add more as experience is gained.

C. Value-Added Time Reporting Log

The Value-Added Time Reporting Log will be utilized to track the process cycle times. This will be ongoing throughout the Lean project. The Log will be forwarded to the manager monthly for further analysis and record keeping. It will provide:

- An accurate, data driven departmental performance indicator
- A current analysis of work loads
- A way to look for continuous improvements ideas
- Data to justify assistance when work volume increases

The Log should be filled out every time that process is started and ended, along with who completed the work. The Log should be placed on the inside front flap of the process folder.

Value-Added Time Reporting Log

Name_____   Date_____

Department_____   Job Title or Function_____

Process Name	Date	Start Time	End Time	Initials	Comments

D. Process Flowchart

A process flowchart is a visual representation of a sequence of activities or tasks that are needed to complete a process. It can be represented by using icons. (See Problem Solving)

Note: Detailed written instructions can also suffice for this step.

3. Establish a holding point.

It is important to create a physical device and place the organizational knowledge (process folders) in a common location.

Note: As you begin to create and collect information about the processes, immediately begin to place the process folders in a common device at a specific location. All of the processes cannot be done at once. The ones that are initially targeted are to be placed in a common area. The process folder will start out in an active state because it contains work that needs to be completed. The process folders should be placed as close to point-of-use as possible.

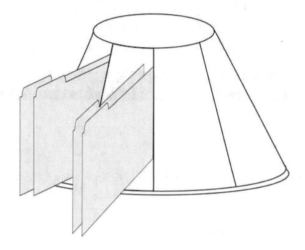

Key Points for the Paper File System in Healthcare

- Start with a good representation of the processes, you will not be able to work on all of them at once.
- Gain a consensus on the critical processes, as they should be the first process folders created.
- Keep the color code simple at first. Do not try to complicate this or you might lose enthusiasm.
- Always work to communicate the need of this system. Emphasize how it will assist in reducing stress by having defined processes and clear standards.
- Continue to recognize the team in their efforts.
- The folder system (and leveling) is critical in obtaining continuous flow for paperwork, take it one step at a time.

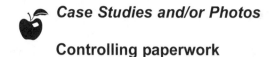

Case Studies and/or Photos

Controlling paperwork

Hospitals still continue to have paperwork. In an effort to improve the visibility and flow of paperwork, consider the following types of examples that utilize the Lean concept in terms of leveling and flow.

This example shows Friday's work (T + 1) as well as Monday's work (T +2). T stands for today, + 1 stands for tomorrow, etc. Friday's and Monday's work have different colored folders (not shown). This system balances the work loads from numerous value streams.

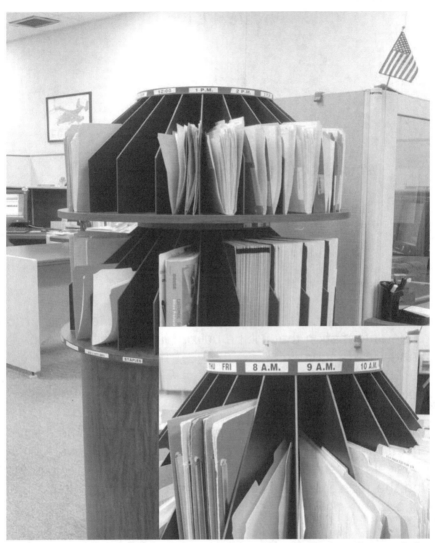

This example shows paperwork that is organized by the hour in an administrative setting. The folders that contain the work are referred to as kanbans. Each kanban contains 60 minutes of work. The bottom right photo shows the folders in their active or passive state. This heijunka box (circular file cabinet) contains three distinct value streams.

Physical Layout

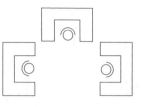

 Why use it?

This will create a self-contained, well-occupied space that optimizes the flow of work, people, and information.

Who does it?

The Lean project team will work with everyone involved to gather information that will be utilized in any facility or departmental rearrangement.

How long will it take?

This should take 2-4 hours to plan. Depending on the degree of rearrangement, it can take an hour to a few days for the physical rearrangement. Be flexible. Conditions may change and the rearrangement may need to be modified after a trial period.

 What does it do?

A new physical layout can accomplish many things, such as:

- Ensure the most efficient layout for the staff and work flow
- Ensure reduction or elimination of excess travel and motion wastes
- Allow for staff flexibility through sharing of work when necessary

- Can be U-shaped, S-shaped, or L- shaped, depending on each work area
- Reduce stress
- Encourage and increase organizational process knowledge versus individual process knowledge

How do you do it?

The six steps to implementing a new physical layout are:

1. Draw a layout of current furniture (i.e., desks, cabinets, nursing stations, charting stations, etc.) as well as common areas (i.e., conference rooms, central supply areas, kitchenettes, etc.).

2. Review the value stream map to determine where wait times are an issue and pose problems.

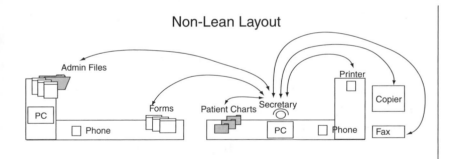

Non-Lean Layout

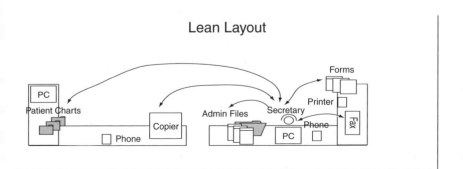

Lean Layout

3. Brainstorm with the team and apply appropriate Lean tools. Determine the most efficient layout. This will reduce transport and motion waste.

4. Create a Standard Work Chart for the new physical layout. (See Standard Work)

5. Implement how work can be delivered to and pulled from the work area. For example, if someone is constantly being requested to fax lab work, then consideration should be given to moving the fax machine closer to that person.

6. Review the new physical layout within 2 weeks after the initial move. Be open to suggestions from staff and be flexible enough to make changes when necessary. Update the Standard Work Chart.

Note: When creating the new physical layout, remember to keep in mind takt times and value stream requirements. Do not create a layout that does not accommodate these.

Key Points for Physical Layout in Healthcare

- Use cross-training to further assist the new layout.
- Keep the continuous flow concept as a focus when designing a new layout.
- Utilize FIFO lanes and In-process supermarkets to assist in the layout.
- Do not create a layout that cannot be changed. If after six months it is working, then permanent resources can be allocated.
- Keep focus on eliminating waste of travel and motion.
- Address staff's concerns over the new arrangement privately.
- Establish before and after measurements to document work flow improvements.

Pitch

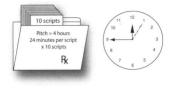

 Why use it?

Pitch establishes a time frame in which consistent and smooth work flow occurs throughout the value stream. It can be a multiple of takt time.

Who does it?

The Lean team will collect data to obtain takt times and establish reasonable pitch. (See Measurement Techniques)

How long will it take?

Plan on spending 1 - 2 hours determining and calculating.

 What does it do?

Pitch is used to reduce wait time between processes or work areas. For example, a medical office found it was constantly calling in prescriptions throughout the day, which was an inefficient use of time. Pitch was used and prescriptions were called in twice a day, which increased the office productivity.

Takt time for many healthcare practices (i.e., blood draws, charting, dispersing medications, etc.) typically will be too small of a unit of time to move the work or information to the next process immediately; therefore, pitch needs to be established to determine the optimal work flow through the value stream. Pitch is the adjusted takt time (or multiple of) when takt time is too short.

Pitch will:

- Set the optimal work flow
- Set the frequency for movement of work and assist in reducing transport and motion waste
- Allow for immediate attention to interruptions of work flow
- Reduce wait times

Note: Each value stream will require a separate pitch. When multiple pitches and value streams are integrated into the department, leveling should be used with a Heijunka or Leveling box. (See Leveling)

Pitch increments must be monitored to ensure they are being met. If an interruption of work arises, a system should be in place to address why the work is behind schedule.

Leveling Box					
Department Lab					
See the Standard Work Chart for how the leveling box operates					
	8:00am	10:00am	1:00pm	3:00pm	
Floors	//	//	//	//	
Clinics	/	/	/	/	
ER/PRN		/		/	

How do you do it?

1. Calculate takt time. (See Takt Time)

2. Determine the optimal number of work units to move through the value stream (i.e., number of labs to be drawn, number of patients to be seen within a specified time period, number of charts to be processed, etc.).

3. Multiply takt time by the optimal number of work units.

Pitch = takt time (x) optimal number of work units

For example:

(1) Prescription request to pharmacy: 20 prescriptions
Time is an 8 hour day (or 480 minutes)
Takt time: Time/Volume = 480 minutes / 20 prescriptions = 24 minutes

(2) Optimal number of prescriptions to be moved = 10 (Ten scripts can easily be called in at one time)

(3) Pitch = 24 minutes x 10 prescriptions = 240 minute pitch or 4 hours

This means every 4 hours, 10 prescriptions will be moved to the next process within the value stream (i.e., the pharmacy).

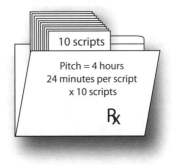

10 scripts

Pitch = 4 hours
24 minutes per script
x 10 scripts

Rx

Key Points for Pitch in Healthcare

- Pitch increments should be created with a visual aid to assist in identifying when interruptions occur (or within a 1 pitch increment).
- Keep pitch increments to at least 2 hours long.
- Make pitch visible to all staff through visual aids (i.e., posters on a wall, signs near the process or work area, etc.) indicating the pitch times.
- Identify interruption resolution procedures if pitch increments cannot be met.
- Adjust pitch increments as patient, staff, or providers demand changes or other issues prevail.
- Create a Standard Work Chart for the pitch process. (See Standard Work)

Case Studies and/or Photos

Phlebotomy

For the morning blood draw, each phlebotomist was expected to draw about 30 patients between 6 and 9 am. However, if they waited until they were done to bring the specimens down to the lab, there would be a delay in the turn-around time for the specimens that were drawn first. The lab calculated their takt time as 180 minutes / 30 patients = 6 minutes. The optimal number to be drawn, before sending the specimens down to the lab, was thought to be 5. Pitch was calculated as 6 minutes (takt time) x 5 specimens (optimal number of work units) = 30 minutes. Therefore, the phlebotomists were asked to send down specimens via the pneumatic tube system every half hour.

Facilities

When beds are changed on the nursing units, the dirty linens are placed in a cart for pick-up. One nursing unit could generate 6 full carts per day, leading to problems if they were left for a single pick-up at the end of the shift. The Facilities Manager worked with the Nursing Director to calculate takt time - in 24 hours, 6 carts were filled, so the takt time = 4 hours. One linen tech could move two carts at a time. Pitch was calculated as 4 hours (takt time) x 2 carts (optimal number of work units) = 8 hours.

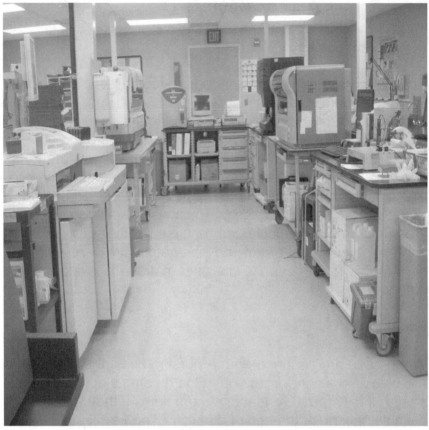

U-shape work areas can assist in meeting pitch times. One operator working multiple instruments situated in a U-shape configuration saves valuable operator's waiting time and reduces unnecessary transportation, while expediting critical testing time. A WIN-WIN scenario for laboratory, clinician, and patient.

Predictable Output

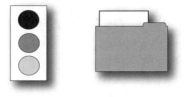

 Why use it?

This creates the expectation of a process which produces a service or work unit with no waste.

Who does it?

The Lean project team will create an awareness on the importance of predictable output. Everyone will work with the Lean tools to obtain predictable output.

How long will it take?

This should take 1-2 hours to plan and merely 10-15 minutes to explain to the team.

What does it do?

Working with repeatable results, based on a consistent process, yields patient, staff, and/or provider satisfaction. That is what predictable output is about. In healthcare, there are no guarantees. Predictable output is not referring to the outcome of the patient's health. It is referring to the processes that provides the needed services.

Predictable output is in our daily lives. The following are processes in society from which we expect predictable output:

- Calling 911 or other emergency services
- Traffic lights
- Using a computer
- Turning on the television
- Turning on/off the lights
- Starting a car

The result of unpredictable output from one of these can range from annoying to deadly. Striving for predictable output from a process is essential for maintaining effective work flow.

How do you do it?

1. Create examples of predictable output that all employees can relate to. Add to the list above.

2. Determine internal errors or interruptions when predictable outcome is not achieved.

3. Communicate the previous two steps to staff. Continually reinforce the concepts of predictable output by:

- Providing relevant examples everyone can relate to
- Providing work related examples as often as possible
- Utilizing standard work to reinforce predictable output

4. Conduct the Predictable Output Survey.

The Predictable Output Survey will provide further understanding of why Lean in healthcare is needed. This can be completed by the manager and shared with the team, or it can be completed as a team exercise for all to understand this basic premise of Lean.

Predictable Output Survey

Name _____   Date _____

Department _____   Job Title or Function _____

The following is a list of questions to further understand current facility practices.	Yes	No
1. Are there standard methods and processes that ensure the quality of work or service?		
2. Are standard methods and processes continually improved upon?		
3. Are standard methods and processes made visible and easily accessible?		
4. Are methods and processes documented?		
5. Do meetings focus on the process and not the personalities?		
6. Are staff involved in a systematic process for improvement?		
7. Is value-added work evenly distributed?		
8. Are staff made aware of Lean tools and concepts?		

If you answer No to any of these, then Lean is needed in your area.

Comments

_____

_____

_____

_____

Please forward to the unit or departmental manager or supervisor when completed.

If you answer "No" to any of these, then Lean is needed in your area. Use the Predictable Output Survey as confirmation of the need for Lean tools.

Predictable output cannot be achieved without standardizing processes. Staff must follow a standardized process that results in a predictable output of a process. This ensures the quality of work is consistent among everyone that must perform to the process. Allowing several different approaches to getting the job done will create only chaos and unpredictability. By developing a best practice for each process, it will be easier to replicate high performance.

Key Points for Predictable Output in Healthcare

- Predictable output cannot be achieved without all staff having a thorough understanding of its importance.
- Predictable output is the foundation for Lean healthcare.
- Create visual aids to relate predictable output to your work area.
- Remember to utilize standard work in establishing predictable output.
- Continually focus on the process of predictable output.
- Use the survey as another tool to communicate the need for Lean in the facility.

Problem Solving

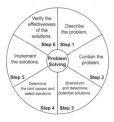

Why use it?

This creates a common language and systematic approach to correcting a deviation from a norm.

Who does it?

Everyone, at all levels of the organization participates.

How long will it take?

It can take anywhere from one hour to several weeks with multiple sessions, depending on the complexity of the problem.

What does it do?

Good problem solving will compliment any Lean initiative. It also:

- Provides the Lean team with an approach to defining the reason(s) for the problem
- Prevents problems from returning
- Creates better standards
- Encourages teamwork

Note: See the Six Sigma section for a more sophisticated problem solving methodology.

The following graph illustrates an event which has occurred causing a negative change in performance. Once a team has identified the event, using the problem solving methodology, they would then be able to increase performance at or above the original level.

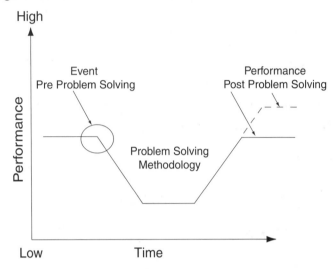

 How do you do it?

The problem solving methodology has several advantages:

- It is simple
- Both groups and individuals can use it
- It can be used at all levels of the organization
- It focuses the team on the issue at hand with minimal training

The six steps to the problem solving methodology are:

1. Describe the problem.
2. Contain the problem.
3. Brainstorm and determine potential solutions.
4. Determine the root causes.
5. Implement the solutions.
6. Verify the effectiveness of the solutions.

THE NEW LEAN HEALTHCARE POCKET GUIDE XL

1. Describe the problem.

This is the crucial step! Approach it as follows:

a. Write a statement describing the problem. A good problem statement describes the situation both in terms of your own experience and measurable terms.

b. The statement should be:
   - Specific - what is it, what is it not? How big is the problem? Is it increasing, decreasing, or unchanging?
   - Time frame - when did it first appear? How was it first identified? Are there co-existing events which impact the problem?
   - Current trend - what is the present situation? Is it increasing, decreasing, or unchanging?

The following is an example of a good problem statement:

"Admissions wait time, identified by the July patient survey, has been increasing from an average of 15 - 20 minutes per patient visit to more than 30 minutes per patient visit during the past six months. The co-existing events are multiple staff retirements and lack of staff replacement."

The following Is/Is Not form can be used to guide the team in problem identification. This form will assist in clarifying what the problem is. It also identifies issues or areas which do not impact or pertain to the current problem.

IS/IS NOT					

Symptom _____ Date _____

Problem Description _____

Is/Is Not Questions	IS	IS NOT	Deductions About Facts		
			Differences	Changes	Date
What Observed					
Where Observed					
When Observed When first observed? When else observed?					
Magnitude How many areas/depts or processes have encountered this problem?					
Trend Increasing or decreasing over time					

2. Contain the problem.

This step is about taking the necessary actions to ensure the patient, provider, or staff does not experience any of the negative effects caused by the problem. It is often a "band-aid" until a permanent solution can be implemented.

The containment may or may not be part of the permanent solution (Step 5).

3. Brainstorm and determine potential solutions.

Once the problem has been identified, and temporarily contained, it is time to analyze the problem carefully.

a. Gather data on the problem.

b. Use one or more of the following analysis tools to assist in this process.

The following ten tools provide a catalyst to help further identify the problem and provide potential solutions.

I. 5 Whys

Most often you will observe a symptom of the problem rather than the problem itself. Always ask "Why?" When answered, each of the 5 Why questions will provide more and more detail about the root cause of the problem.

Problem Statement: Admissions wait time, identified by the July patient survey, has been increasing from an average of 15-20 minutes per patient visit to more than 30 minutes per patient visit during the past six months. The co-existing events are multiple staff retirements and lack of staff replacement.

Why?
Lack of staff.

Why?
2 early retirements.

Why?
Lack of replacement staff.

Why?
The reallocation of resources.

Why?
Budget constraints.

II. Flowcharts or process maps

Creating a flowchart or process map allows for a visual representation of a sequence of activities or tasks consisting of people, work duties, and transactions that occur for the delivery of a product or service. It is one of the most effective methods to document a process.

When creating a flowchart, the project team should approach the activity like an investigation. The team should find out exactly what is happening and what is not happening in the process. The following symbols can be utilized in creating a process map:

Begin or End - represents the initial start or end of a process

Activity or Step - represents the various tasks within a process

Decision - represents an alternative process flow given some type of criteria

Flow - represents the direction of activity flow

Wait time - represents a delay in the process

Document - represents a form, worksheet, or computer file that needs to be completed

Protocol - represents a standard to follow (i.e., standards of service, standard operating procedure, etc.)

Connection - represents continuation to the next process or page

Note: These are the standard set of flowchart icons. The team can create news ones if that would assist in improving the visualization of process flow.

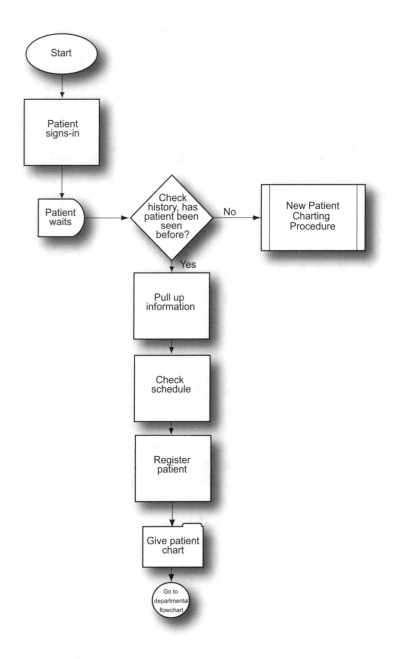

III. Frequency Charts and Check Sheets

Frequency Charts, also referred to as Check Sheets, are used to collect, organize, prioritize, and analyze data. They can be used to answer the question, "How often is an event occurring?" They help you track activities.

Frequency Chart		
Department Admissions	Start Date_____	End Date_____
Task #	Task Name	Frequency of Task
1	Answering phones	||
2	Faxing	|||
3	Entering patient demographics	||||
4	Updating schedules	ⅥⅢ ||
5	Calling for information	|||
6	Billing	|

IV. Cause & Effect or Fishbone Diagrams

Cause & Effect Diagrams (also referred to as Fishbone Diagrams) are used to clearly show the various factors affecting a process. This is done by identifying the problem on the right side of the diagram, then by brainstorming and data collection listing potential causes of the problem on the left side of the diagram. The left side is used to identify and prioritize all causes. If done properly and completely, the cause of the problem is somewhere on the diagram.

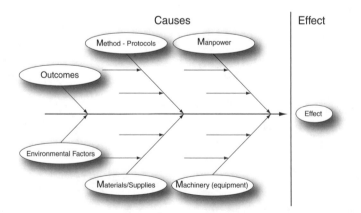

130

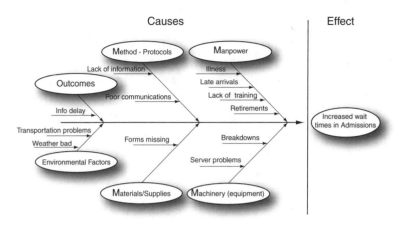

V. Pareto Charts

The Pareto Chart is a type of bar chart used in problem identification. It lists the issues in descending order of importance. These charts are used to prioritize and break down complex problems into smaller sections. They also help to identify multiple root causes by looking at the highest percentage of involvement. When the major categories are identified and dealt with, the other categories are often resolved.

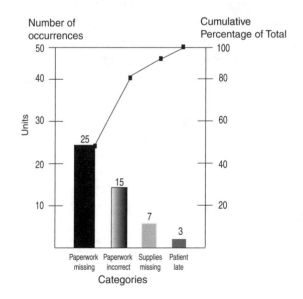

VI. Histograms

Histograms utilize measurement data and display the spread and shape of the distribution. They are a simple graphical representation for the dimensional performance of a sample of data. A histogram is a "picture" of the sample data. Histograms only provide a clue as to how the process is running.

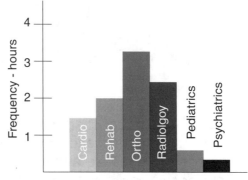

Units - Type of Care - Emergency

VII. Control Charts

Control Charts are basically line graphs plotted over a specified time period. The vertical axis contains the quantitative measurement of the problem, while the horizontal axis is based on a time interval. There are many variations of control charts. Control Charts are very useful for tracking progress over time.

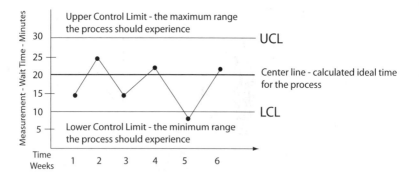

VIII. Scatter and Concentration Plots

Scatter and Concentration Plots are used to study the possible relationship between one variable and another.   Through visual examination and additional mathematical analysis, relationships between variables can be determined.

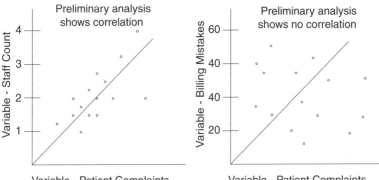

IX. Brainstorming

Brainstorming is used to capture people's ideas and organize those thoughts around common themes (or the identified problem).   During brainstorming sessions there should be no criticism of anyone's ideas.   You are trying to open possibilities and break down incorrect assumptions about the problem.

Let people have fun brainstorming.   Encourage them to come up with as many ideas as possible.   Encourage creativity.

When brainstorming, ensure that no train of thought is followed for too long.   Ideas generated from the brainstorming session should be evaluated while exploring potential solutions to the problem.

X. Storyboarding

The Storyboard is typically a poster-size framework for holding all key information. It is a visual aid for a problem solving or Lean project. The Storyboard is organized into various areas that can be represented by a graph, illustration, and/or a simple sentence or two. The information is then displayed on a format that is graphically rich and engaging. The Storyboard will contain many problem solving (or Lean) tools representing the problem solving process.

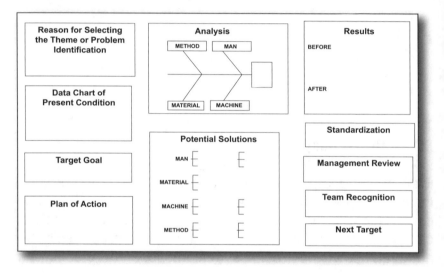

4. Determine the root causes and select solutions.

Root cause is the deep underlying cause of a problem in a process or system. Many of the tools explained in the previous section can also be used to assist in determining the root cause. Each potential root cause must be tested to ensure a permanent solution is implemented.

Clarify what constraints might apply to a proposed solution (required approvals, timing, impact on other departments, etc.). The following statements may be useful in determining root cause(s):

- You ran out of ideas when asking, "What caused the problem to begin with?"
- All conversation has halted and everyone is confident that the root cause(s) has been identified
- Everyone connected to the problem believes the root cause can be eliminated now
- The root cause seems logical and there is no confusion
- Finding the root cause(s) has given staff hope that something positive can be done to prevent reoccurrence of the problem
- Agreement is reached concerning workable solutions

5. Implement the solutions.

Gain a consensus on the action plan. Ensure key decision makers approve the course of action. Plan the implementation: when will it start, who will be doing what, and what types of measurements will be utilized.

6. Verify the effectiveness of the solutions.

Once implementation has begun, ensure the correct measurements are in place. Track each solution relative to the problem description. If the problem has been eliminated, update the work standards or documentation.

If the problem has not improved to the team's satisfaction, return to Step 1. Learn from this experience. Do not go down the same path.

After each step, use the Problem Solving Storyboard to consolidate the project as it is occurring and as a final report.

Problem Solving Storyboard	
Department _____	**Start Date** _____
Team Name	**Team Members**
#1 Describe the problem. SYMPTOM	**#2 Contain the problem.**
#3 Brainstorm and determine the solutions. Phase Completion Date:_____	
#4 Determine the root causes and select solutions. CAUSE Phase Completion Date:_____	
#5 Implement the solutions. REMEDY	**#6 Verify the effectiveness of the solutions.** Phase Completion Date:_____

Key Points for Problem Solving in Healthcare

- Use the quick-fixes (band-aids) for containing the problem and then continue with all steps.
- Step 1 is the most important step in the process.
- Most failures in problem solving are a result of jumping to conclusions.

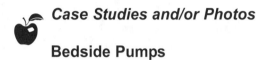

Case Studies and/or Photos

Bedside Pumps

Following surgery, many patients have pumps at their bedside for the administration of narcotics. One hospital had one key per floor that controlled all the pumps. There was no set location for the key. Whichever nurse used the key last usually had it in his or her pocket. Whenever a nurse needed to refill the medication or change the drug dosage, he or she would have to go and search for the key. The patient had to wait for his or her medication. Looking at this process from a Lean problem solving perspective, much of nursing time was being spent trying to find the nurse with the key. The activity of searching for the key was identified as being non value-added and the root cause of the problem. The new process had multiple keys being issued, one for each nurse per shift per unit (floor or ward). At the end of each shift, a key was passed from one nurse to the other. A form was signed by both nurses indicating transfer of the key. Four years later, the nurses are happier and no keys have been lost. This resulted in the following outcomes:

1. Decreased nurse frustration and increased nurse satisfaction
2. Decreased waste of motion for the nursing staff
3. Shortened the lead time of pump adjustments and medication administration
4. Increased patient satisfaction by making necessary medications immediately available

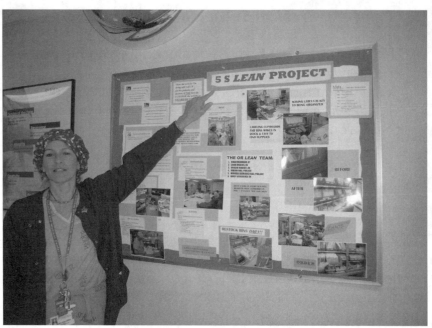

Storyboards should be located in a common location. Storyboards can be an effective communication tool.

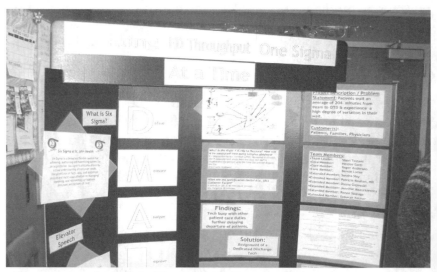

The Storyboard is titled, "Tracking ED Throughput One Sigma At a Time" and was on display at an organizational learning day. This learning day brought together improvement projects from numerous hospitals.

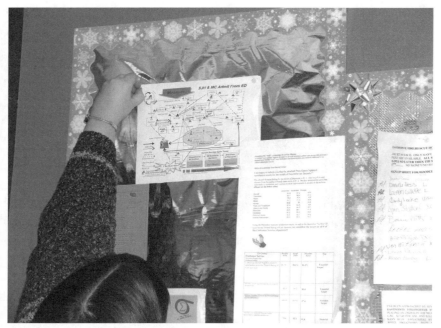

Storyboards should be updated on a regular basis as the team progresses throughout the improvement project.

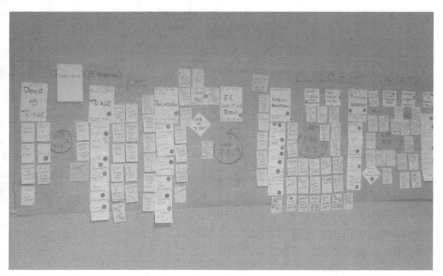

Good problem solvign begins with a detailed understanding of the current state.

Pull Systems

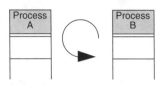

 Why use it?

This will create a system in which nothing is produced by an upstream supplier process until the downstream customer process signals the need for it. This enables work to flow without detailed schedules. It is the opposite of Push, where work is completed and passed downstream regardless of need or request. For example, central supply replenishes the supplies requested from the various floors and departments only when they are needed, not automatically.

Who does it?

The Lean project team will utilize the Lean tools and create the pull system. Everyone in the value stream will contribute to improving the system once it is in place.

How long will it take?

This will depend on the complexity of the value stream, number of processes connected, and the variety of work being completed. The Lean project team must spend 2-4 hours on each value stream to analyze how a pull system can be implemented. Implementation may take 1-2 weeks to complete. And then ongoing improvements as required.

What does it do?

To create a Pull System there needs to be a very good (data rich) understanding of the downstream process(es).

The Pull System is based on a signal (i.e., kanban) used to inform an upstream process that work is required. This signal will prevent the overproduction of work (waste) and ensure only what is required downstream will be produced. A true Pull System is a challenge in administrative areas due to the variability in customer demand at the downstream process. Therefore, the tools of FIFO and In-process supermarkets are utilized. (See Continuous Flow)

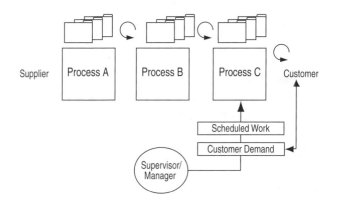

There are two types of kanbans:

The withdrawal kanban is a printed card, folder, email alert, pager code, flag, light, etc., used as a visual aid indicating the quantity of work to be removed from the In-process supermarket. (See Paper File System)

A production kanban is a printed card, folder, email alert, pager code, flag, light, etc., used as a visual aid indicating what is required to be processed from a downstream request (or from the In-process supermarket). (See Paper File System)

Note: Do not get caught up in the different types. A kanban simply is a signal initiated by a downstream process to trigger work or a service to be completed by an upstream process.

How do you do it?

1. Learn the tools of kanbans, FIFO, and In-process supermarkets.

2. Gather appropriate downstream data from the process(es). Include cycle times, number of interruptions, and volume of work for a specified value stream.

3. Brainstorm with the team to see how a Pull System can be utilized.

4. Create the appropriate visual aids; either kanban cards or another type of visual control, to signal a work request or to indicate not to produce more work.

5. Create a Standard Work Chart. (See Standard Work)

6. Train staff to the new system.

7. Implement the system and work towards improvements.

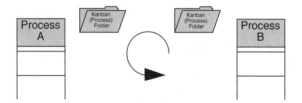

For example: The billing office of a medical clinic may request, via e-mail, a certain number of Patient Encounter Forms to be processed. The request would be triggered by the down-stream process (billing) to have the upstream process (clinical department) only send what can be processed within a certain time.

Key Points for Pull Systems in Healthcare

- Kanbans are a signal to inform an upstream process that it can release work or provide additional service to the downstream process.
- Kanbans are the heart of the Pull System.
- Kanbans should be a standard card, folder, e-mail, pager code, etc.
- No upstream process should release the kanban unless it is error-free.
- Kanbans always travel with the work to ensure Just-In-Time information and provide a visual control.

Case Studies and/or Photos

Medicine Unit

Nurses on a Medicine unit were very frustrated. They had recently experienced several "near misses" when an IV pump was almost used for a patient, only to find out it had not been cleaned after the previous use. And, they were spending a lot of time searching for commodes and other items. This had a big impact on the time nurses could spend on patient care.

The Nurse Manager asked them to help come up with a better way to deal with their equipment. The nurses agreed to keep track of equipment issues for a week, including time spent searching, and noting which items were problems. They made up a data collection form and agreed to place completed forms in a special "IN BOX." The data collection was done over one week, and then was collated by the Nurse Manager, to be shared at the next unit meeting.

At the next unit meeting, the results showed that there were 5 items requiring BioMed processing and 25 minor supply items had been searched for during the previous week. The time spent searching or dealing with equipment issues averaged 75 minutes per nurse on days and 90 minutes on nights.

The Nurse Manager asked a small team to get together to determine a) which items had the greatest impact of time lost; b) how many items were needed of those, ready on the unit, per day; and c) a process for making sure that they had the items they needed, when they needed them.

The team worked with the BioMed department to identify space in the clean and the dirty utility room, where the key items would be placed - they taped off areas for each group of items, on the floor and on the shelves, in both rooms. They identified the maximum and minimum number for each item, according to how many would be needed for a typical day, plus an additional amount for a "buffer." The process included:

BioMed using a green label to identify a "clean" or "ready" item, which would be removed when placed into use; a designated "minimum" and "maximum" amount of each item; a phone call to BioMed when the minimum number was reached; a promise to BioMed to respond by bringing up clean/ready items and taking away the dirty items for processing. For supplies, the person taking the item from the storage area, that would bring the items to the minimum count, would follow the directions to obtain more. These directions were posted after getting agreement from BioMed and the Materials Management department.

After two-week trial period, the nurses repeated the data collection exercise to see whether there was a difference. This time they found that day and night Nurses averaged only 15 minutes per shift on equipment-related issues. BioMed gave the unit feedback that their process was working so well, they wanted to implement it in the rest of the hospital.

The unit decided to sustain the gains by doing a "spot monitor" monthly, where nurses would collect one day's worth of observations, and any issues would be discussed at unit meetings. BioMed bought the unit staff pizza and pop to say thanks for making their lives easier and reducing the number of "stat" calls to BioMed for needed equipment.

The results after three months were:

1. Reduction in "near misses" from an average of 6 per month, to 1 per month.
2. Decrease in stat calls to BioMed, from a high of 75 per month to 6 per month.
3. Decrease in BioMed overtime, equating to a cost of $1,250 per month ($15,000 annually).
4. Improved efficiency of nurses and increased time at the bedside; reflected in the decrease from 80 min avg overall per nurse, to 15 min avg overall per nurse (estimated $208,000 annually at average cost for nursing time per hour).

Reporting and Communications

Why use it?

This section is about documentation of Lean initiatives. It is imperative for Lean projects to have the proper flow of communications to all those concerned. The main focus is people's time.

Who does it?

1. The team leader is responsible for the distribution of the various communication tools.

2. The Lean project team is responsible for contributing to and following the formal meeting procedures.

How long will it take?

The Team Charter takes about 1 - 2 hours to prepare. The Meeting Information Form takes about 15 minutes to prepare. The Status Report takes about 5 minutes to prepare.

What does it do?

Proper communication is the basis for continuous improvement. It provides the following:

- Standardizes communications
- Ensures strategic alignment
- Ensures team discipline
- Reduces team meetings
- Reduces stress

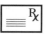 ### *How do you do it?*

There are three forms required to effectively communicate Lean project information.

1. The Team Charter
2. The Meeting Information Form
3. The Status Report

1. Team Charter

The Team Charter is a document detailing the team's mission and deliverable (or outcome) to ensure strategic alignment.

a. The Team Charter is to be completed by the Lean project team assigned to the area requiring improvement. It must be approved by the team champion. The champion is the person that has authority to commit resources from the facility.

b. Completing the Team Charter is the first step in any Lean project. It ensures everyone is on the same page.

c. The Team Charter is a living document and will require updating as conditions change. It should be posted in a common area.

d. The Team Charter will list goals and outcomes.

e. The Lean project team should gain a consensus on the Team Charter and be aware of "scope creep." Scope creep is losing focus on the goal, while at the same time expanding the Lean project area beyond the initial plan.

f. The champion must ensure proper resources are committed. The champion usually does not attend all of the meetings, other than the kick-off meeting. He or she is available to remove roadblocks, break down departmental barriers, and provide any other support.

g. The team leader is responsible for the day-to-day or week-to-week activities. He or she will schedule meetings and inform the champion of progress via Status Reports.

h. The Activity Section will list the broader actions required throughout the duration of the project. (The Meeting Information Form will list the detailed steps of the project.)

i. The facilitator is a person who has no vested interest in the project and will keep the team focused at the meetings.

j. The scribe is a person who will take notes during the meetings.

k. Steering Body Members are typically used for larger projects. They would be comprised of members from the Board of Directors, Chief Medical Officer, Clinical Nurse Manager, Chief Financial Officer, Facility's Manager, etc. Smaller projects would utilize only the team champion.

Team Charter

Mission

The team will evaluate the Emergency Department process from "Dispo" to "Admit." This is from the time the physician determines that the patient needs to be admitted to the time the patient is placed in his/her inpatient bed and all hand-offs have been completed.

Outcomes

The team will create a streamlined process flow to achieve the following:
Reduce ED LOS for Dispo-to-Admit approx. 50% (from 170 mins to 90 mins)
Reduce ED LOS for Admit Patients by 25% (from 360 mins to 270 mins)
Improve ED (Patient) Satisfaction score by 50%

Deliverables

1. Create a current and future state value stream map of the ED patient experience.
2. Create and implement new standard work for the process of Dispo-to-Admit.
3. Create a Failure Prevention Analysis Worksheet to ensure mistake proofing of any process change.
4. Train all staff on new standards. Implement a 5S program throughout the ED.
5. Monitor changes (and adjust if necessary) to ensure changes are controlled and sustained over time.

Expected Scope/Approach/Activities

1. The scope of the team's authority and focus is: ED processes between physician order to admit and patient being placed into the bed. Changes to be approved during the event by the Process Owner, ED Manager, and Bed Placement Coordinator, with communication/training for other stakeholders as appropriate.
2. The approach will use the Value Stream Management methodology to achieve the deliverables.
3. In addition to the week-long focused Kaizen Event, the team will conduct preparatory meetings as needed to support the Event week, including contacting IT and facilities for expected support during the Event week.

Strategic Alignment Factors

- ED LOS for Admitted Patients
- Efficiency (decreased time in the ED places pt more quickly in less costly care on the in patient unit)
- Growth (opening capacity and decreasing "Left Without Being Seen" for other patients)
- Clinical Effectiveness (care by the ED physician is focused on immediate conditions, while care by the admitting physician is focused on the patient's short and long term needs)

Team Process

Process Item	Frequency	Audience/Distribution
Stakeholder Check	• Daily, during, and 30-60-90 day post-Event	• Team members, face-to-face, for all stakeholders
Information Distribution	• Once, after first preparatory meetings • Daily, after each day of the Event • 30-60-90 day follow-up	• From team to stakeholders, after first preparatory meeting • From team to entire hospital staff
Team Meetings	• Three prep meetings in three weeks prior • Daily, during the Event, weekly follow-ups	• Team, Process Owner, Fac., Champion • Team, Process Owner, Facilitator
Status Reporting	• 30-60-90 Follow-up reports	• Team, Process Owner, Fac., Champion

Expected Results

Benefits (What results will be gained?)	Metrics (How will the results be measured?)
1. Reduced cycle time, Dispo-to-Admit by 45% (est) 2. Improved ED Patient Satisfaction by 50+%	1. Cycle time metrics collected weekly 2. Patient Satisfaction scores, weekly mean scores

Assumptions

- ED patient volumes will remain consistent
- ED staffing will support change

Risks

- ED staff will not follow new standards
- Some stakeholders will not support change

Internal Issues

- ED physicians not engaged after admit order written
- Disagreement among physicians who should write order
- Staffing concerns with nursing
- Nurse Planning may relieve staff on units due to low census

External Issues

- Joint Commission's new requirements on patient hand-offs and transportation between units

LAN Location/Revision #	**Facility Confidential**

2. Meeting Information Form

The Meeting Information Form provides the team with a structured approach to effective meetings, including detailed agendas and action items.

a. The Meeting Information Form should be created and forwarded by the team leader to team members at least 24 hours prior to the meeting and within 24 hours after the meeting has concluded.

b. Action times/due dates are assigned and reviewed at the meetings. Every attempt is made to adhere to the dates agreed to when assigning action items.

c. List the status of action items as closed or open.

d. The agenda should be detailed enough (usually 5 minute increments) to indicate the time allocated for the various segments of the meeting time.

Meeting Information Form

Logistics

Meeting Title:	ED Arrival to Inpatient Bed Team Kick-off
Date:	4/3
Time:	1300 - 1530
Place:	ED Conference Room
Purpose:	Review Team Charter and set goals for improvement project

Distribution / FYI Copies

Participants	Roles	Stakeholders	Roles
Bill, Anne, Sarah, John, Randy, and Dr. Ben	Core team members	VPs, Execs	Support
Sue R.	Facilitator - Trainer		
Margaret S.	Process Owner/ Team Leader		
Mary H., Judy D.	Co-Champions		

Agenda

Time	Item	Who	Duration (minutes)
1300	Icebreaker, purpose of meeting, strategic direction, commitment from execs	J.A./M.H.	15
1315	Review Team Charter and Balanced Scorecard	M.H./M.S.	30
1345	Introduction to Lean, high level review of VSM	S.R.	60
1445	Introduction to healthcare waste (activity)	S.R./M.S.	30
1515	Determine tasks, schedule next meeting	S.R./M.S.	15
1530	Depart	All	

Action Items (to be completed by next meeting or sooner)

No.	Action Item	Who	Start Date	End Date	Status
1	Create VOC survey	S.S.	4/3	4/10	Open
2	Gather data for processes within ED	B.H.	4/3	4/10	Open
3	Gather benchmark data	J.L.	4/3	4/10	Open

LAN Location/Revision #   **Confidential**

3. Status Report

The Status Report communicates the progress to date.

a. The Status Report should be created and forwarded to the champion every two weeks (or weekly) by the team leader.

b. The Status Report must include potential resolutions for any problems or concerns listed.

c. The Status Report should not take the place of one-on-one communications with the team champion.

Status Report

Team Name   ED Arrival to Inpatient Bed Improvement Team

Date   4/3

Status

(Are you on schedule?)
Yes. The team had one meeting as planned to align theTeam Charter with
the Balanced Scoreard and ED Goal Card. A brief overview of Lean, as well as
a review of wastes in healthcare, was completed.
The team agreed to have weekly meetings to further analyze and plan for the
improvements for the Dispo-to-Admit portion of the Level I value stream.
The second week in May was scheduled for the Kaizen Event week.
The detailed timeline for the tasks can be found at
www.oakview.org/ED_DispoVSM_Timeline.

Accomplishments

Everyone was in attendance for the first meeting.

Concerns (Issues)

None at present. Future concerns may include how to train staff on new process;
possible resistance by physicians; and, how to accelerate approvals for form
changes.

Plans (How to Resolve Issues)

Stakeholders will be communicated to on regular basis per the team's mission
and timetable.

LAN Location/Revision #1   **Facility Confidential**

Key Points for Reporting and Communications in Healthcare

- It is helpful to have the Team Charter semi-completed prior to the first Lean team meeting. This may save some time in presenting the core information.
- The Team Charter is a living document and should reflect the team's input as it is periodically reviewed and updated.
- The team leader should always prepare an agenda for a meeting. If a Kaizen Event is going to consume more than a few hours, then the team should detail the specific activities as much as possible.
- The Meeting Information Form can be quickly completed and distributed to all appropriate staff. It is a clear and concise document that communicates what is going on and the individual assignments of the team members.
- Review action items at the start and end of each meeting. If some action items have not been completed on schedule, determine the reason and work with the team or individual in assisting with completion of these items.
- Initially keep all Lean projects to less than 90 days. Reward the team to further promote Lean initiatives.

Resistance to Change

The 80/20 Rule

 Why use it?

This will help you understand why and how people oppose changes, including improvements. Resistance can greatly impact a Lean or Six Sigma project.

Who does it?

The manager/supervisor must take the lead in understanding change. It can be addressed through good communication, education, and co-worker support.

How long will it take?

This should take 2-4 hours to understand and prepare a presentation for the team. The first couple meetings of a Lean project team will determine the resistance that needs to be addressed. Appropriate time should be allocated by the manager/supervisor to privately talk with those people who are resisting the change(s).

What does it do?

Understanding the resistance to change will allow for clearer communications. Change is inevitable. Most resistance is due to the lack of communication and understanding. Staff may not know how the change (or improvements) will affect them. Use the Ultimate Case Studies for Lean in Healthcare and Predictable Output sections of *The New Lean Healthcare Pocket Guide XL* to address the overall need for change.

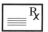 ### *How do you do it?*

Overcoming resistance to change involves four steps.

1. Understand the 4 S's of resistance.
2. Analyze "quick adapters."
3. Apply the 80/20 rule.
4. Conduct a meeting.

1. Understand the 4 S's of resistance.

Resistance to Skills
Resistance to Support
Resistance to Society
Resistance to Stress

Resistance to Skills is due to the increase in anxiety of new work requirements that may appear too technical, too complicated, or require skills that a staff member may or may not have. The easiest and most effective way to address this fear is to provide employees with information, training, and education. This will prepare them to master the skills required to implement the changes. Resistance to Lean Healthcare will most likely occur. Lean requires a different, more efficient way of doing things.

Resistance to Support is due to people understanding that as new processes are streamlined, their jobs may be at risk. In some cases this may be a justifiable fear. Some job functions will change and some departments will be consolidated. But as facilities deploy the Lean tools, they will be in a better position for growth and will then have the ability to shift people to other functions. Acknowledge the difficulty this presents to the employee. Empathize with the employees' concern of the changes that may affect them. Point out the benefits of Lean as a long term solution for job security, advancement, and organizational growth.

Resistance to Society is due to some people being resistant to *any* ideas that do not originate with them. Their pride and ego won't let them accept any idea that does not have their "stamp" on it. Fortunately, implementing Lean tools and practices is a team effort. There are many opportunities for everyone to provide input into how these new systems and procedures are developed and deployed.

Resistance to Stress is due to the variety of difficult challenges the staff may be facing, not only in the office, but in their personal lives as well. If an employee is not making the transition well, the manager/supervisor should quickly find out what the problem is. It may be related to outside stresses not controlled by the organization. In these situations, it is important to understand the personal situation affecting the work. Emphasize and create realistic expectations for the acceptance to the proposed changes.

2. Analyze "quick adapters."

Recognize employees who are leaders. They are present in any workplace. Managers and supervisors must be on the lookout for these leaders. When they are identified, utilize their skills wisely. They could be appointed the day-to-day champion (the person responsible for the Lean project), which will make the Lean healthcare journey easier. Remember, no change can be effective and sustained without employees who have the vision, desire, and willingness to see it through.

There are five levels of support (or lack of) usually found within an organization going through change. They are:

- People who will make it happen
- People who will help it happen
- People who will let it happen
- People who are mildly against it
- People who will actively sabotage it

---

3. Apply the 80/20 rule.

Usually no more than 20% of the employees will fall into the last two categories. Of that 20%, 80% of those people can be converted into supporters, while 20% may never accept any change. Mathematically, $0.8 + (0.8 \times 0.2) = 0.96$, or 96% will be in support. Focus on the 96%!

4. Conduct a meeting.

Conduct a meeting with your group of employees to address the changes and any fears they may have. Continue to monitor progress and acceptance to change.

Key Points for Resistance to Change in Healthcare

- Continue to assure employees of the organization's need to improve. The benefits of a profitable organization will position it for growth while providing job security.
- Continually look for ways to involve staff in the change process.
- Find those informal, day-to-day champions, and utilize them wisely.
- Ensure reward and recognition are used for team and individual contributions.
- Create visual aids about the changes well in advance (i.e., posters, notices, storyboards, etc.).
- Prior to any changes, educate everyone impacted by the proposed changes.

Runners

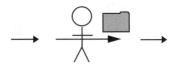

 Why use it?

This will ensure takt time or pitch is maintained, which keeps the focus on value-added activities.

Who does it?

The appointed person is assigned to distribute work to designated areas. This includes value-added activities within the value stream.

How long will it take?

Initially, it will take about 1 hour to brainstorm with the team to determine the runner's role.

 What does it do?

The runner allows for:

- Processes or areas to focus on value-added activities
- A pace of work to be established throughout the day
- Supports service between departments to improve work flow
- Increased productivity

How do you do it?

1. Study the future state process or value stream map. (See Value Stream Mapping)

2. Determine the runner's route with the established pitch time to eliminate waste of transport and motion.

3. Create standard work for the route. (See Standard Work)

Standard Work Chart

Routine Food Tray Delivery		
Process Name	Dietary Department Bulletin Board	
Dietary	Posted Location	
Department		

Takt Time N/A	Upstream Process Name	Downstream Process Name
Pitch - every 4 hours	Food Preparation	Patients Rooms Floor's 2 and 3

Standard Work Sequence for: Runner	Pitch Increment 4 hours - See Schedule
1. Runner departs on a schedule.	
2. Runner picks up menus from nurses station and delivers food trays.	
3. Runner proceeds to north wall for additional menus.	
4. Runner separates menus.	
5. Runner delivers menus to the Dietary In-Basket.	

XOXO

Food Prep

Nurses station

Dietary In

North wall

4. Determine who the runner should be. The following are attributes of a good runner:

- Trained well in value stream requirements
- Good communicator
- Understands Lean concepts
- Understands the importance of takt time and pitch
- Is efficient and effective in work duties
- Has a good attitude toward change

5. Create a runner's cart or carry-all for the work to be held in. Make it as small and versatile as possible.

6. Train the runner and backup runner(s).

7. Monitor the route and update standard work as improvements are suggested.

Key Points for Runners in Healthcare

- A runner must:
  - communicate well
  - see and report problems as they occur
  - understand Lean concepts
  - strive to maintain pitch
  - look for ways to improve the route
- Runners are critical in providing information about the process that is being run. This can assure small problems throughout the day do not become larger ones.
- Runners should have procedures for communicating interruptions when pitch cannot be maintained. For example, the runner may use some type of 3G communication device (cell phone, pager, text message, etc.) to communicate the interruption to the unit manager.

Six Sigma

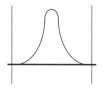

Why use it?

Six Sigma is a sophisticated problem solving approach for improving business performance. Six Sigma is "management driven by data." It is based upon improving processes by controlling and understanding variation, thus improving predictability of business processes. It is a disciplined, data-driven, decision-making methodology.

Note: Six Sigma is an advanced tool and should be used after implementing other Lean tools first.

In its purest form, Six Sigma is a term used to describe a measure of quality control that is near perfection. The Six Sigma Process uses data and rigorous statistical analysis to identify "defects" in a process, service, or product, reduce variability, and achieve as close to zero defects as possible.

Six Sigma is desperately needed in the healthcare system. The healthcare system is far from the zero defect rate. Less than Six Sigma is not good enough because we would have to accept the following in the U.S.:

- 20,000 incorrect drug prescriptions per year
- 500 incorrect surgical operations per week
- 50 newborn babies dropped at birth per day

Who does it?

The Six Sigma process should be facilitated by a Black Belt trained staff member. Achieving Black Belt certification signifies that the individual has successfully completed an improvement activity with a defined cost savings.

How long will it take?

Six Sigma team projects typically will take 1 to 3 months (or longer) depending on the complexity of the problem.

What does it do?

Six Sigma provides the facility with the following:

- Improved patient satisfaction
- Improved productivity of staff
- Improved staff problem solving skills
- Reduced costs
- Reduced number of errors or mistakes
- A standard continuous improvement methodology
- A fact-based decision making process
- A common language throughout the facility

Six Sigma is most effective when used as part of a business improvement strategy. When combined with the philosophy and methods of Lean, it becomes a powerful method for continuous improvement.

Six Sigma is a reference to the goal of reducing defects or mistakes to zero. Sigma is the Greek letter mathematicians used to represent the "standard deviation of a population." The standard deviation of a population represents the variability within a group of items, i.e., the population.

Six Sigma is a measure of variation that achieves 3.4 defects per million opportunities, or 99.99966 percent acceptable. It is represented by the following bell shaped curve. The higher the sigma value, the better.

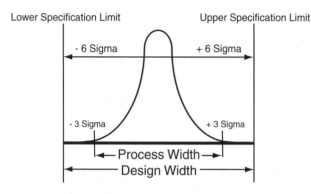

How do you do it?

Six Sigma uses a five step problem solving tool called **D-M-A-I-C**:

1. **D**efine
2. **M**easure
3. **A**nalyze
4. **I**mprove
5. **C**ontrol

1. Define

Define the customers, their requirements, the Team Charter, and the key process that affects the customer. The following tools can be utilized:

- Team Charter
- Process Mapping
- Cause and Effect Diagram
- Affinity Diagram
- Voice of the Customer (VOC) Table

(See Problem Solving for many of these tools)

2. Measure

Identify the key measures and the data collection plan for the process in question. Execute the plan for data collection. The following tools can be utilized:

- Document Tagging
- Data Collection and Check Sheet

(See Data Collection and Document Tagging)

3. Analyze

Analyze the data collected, as well as the process, to determine the root cause(s) for why the process is not performing as desired. The following tools can be utilized:

- Histogram
- Pareto
- Scatter Diagram
- Control or Run Chart
- Design of Experiments (DOE)

(See Problem Solving for many of these tools)

4. Improve

Generate and determine potential solutions and plot them on a small scale to determine if they positively improve process performance. The following tools can be utilized:

- Process Mapping or Flowcharting
- Paynter Chart

(See Problem Solving for many of these tools)

5. Control

Develop, document, and implement a plan to ensure perform-ance improvement remains at the desired level. The following tools can be utilized:

- Control or Run Charts
- Paynter Chart

(See Problem Solving and Standard Work)

The following is an example of how to calculate the Six Sigma capability for one of your processes:

Six Sigma Calculation Worksheet

Process Name Order Entry   **Date**   2/16

No.	Action	Equations	Your Calculations
1	What process do you want to consider?		Order Entry
2	How many units were put through the process?		1,283
3	Of those that went through, how many passed?		1,138
4	Compute the yield for the process	= (Step 3) / (Step 2)	.887
5	Compute the defect rate based on Step 4	= 1 - (Step 4)	.113
6	Determine the number of potential things that could create a defect (note: use N = 10 as a conservative number of potential defects)	= N number of critical-to-quality characteristics (CTQs)	10
7	Compute the defect rate per CTQ characteristic	= (Step 5) / (Step 6)	.0113
8	Compute the defects per million opportunities (DPMO)	= (Step 7) x 1,000,000	11,300
9	Convert the DPMO (Step 8) into a sigma value, using a Six Sigma Conversion Chart (google: six sigma conversion table)	Includes a 1.5 sigma shift for all listed values of Z	3.8
10	Draw conclusions		Opportunity for improvement

Key Points for Six Sigma in Healthcare

- Train employees in the problem solving tools through using healthcare examples as much as possible.
- Utilize a Black Belt for guidance in all phases.
- Use Six Sigma within an overall business improvement strategy.
- Recognize and reward staff as Six Sigma projects are completed.

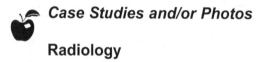

Case Studies and/or Photos

Radiology

The director of a Radiology department discovered that out-patient CT scans were being scheduled three weeks out. This had been increasing over the past six months. Patients were being referred to other facilities - costing the facility the potential revenue of over $30,000 per month.

A multi-disciplinary team was formed and facilitated by a Six Sigma Black Belt. Team members were trained in the principles of Lean and Six Sigma. The team met weekly for 1 - 2 hours, depending on the agenda.

A Team Charter was created with expected outcomes of a 10% reduction in the actual cycle time for the process, as well as reducing the lead time by 50%. The team met for nearly 6 six weeks and used process mapping, cause and effect, check sheets, pareto diagrams, run charts, standard work, and control charts throughout the D-M-A-I-C process.

The team achieved a 17% reduction of overall cycle time for the CT scanning process, increased patient satisfaction due to the decreased wait time, and increased physician satisfaction due to earlier reading of the CT results. This resulted in an earlier diagnosis and treatment for the patient.

Standard Work

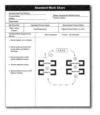

Why use it?

Standard work establishes the best way to do work and/or provide a service. It should be the *basis* for all continuous improvement activities.

Who does it?

The Lean project team will determine best practices, document them, train everyone to those practices, and provide a system for future improvement. Everyone eventually will contribute improvement ideas through the use of standard work.

How long will it take?

Most critical processes for a department or value stream can be identified in a 1-2 hour meeting. Subsequent documentation may take 4 or more hours - depending on the complexity of the process(es). For example, creating standard work for the process of prepping an OR patient would take longer than creating standard work for the process of how to change a dressing.

What does it do?

It establishes the best practice or best sequence of activities, which minimizes waste. Standard work consists of a set of procedures that dictate activities that are always executed consistently with no variation. Standard work is a major component of kaizen activities.

Standard work utilizes two main tools: the Standard Work Combination Table and the Standard Work Chart.

The Standard Work Combination Table will:

- Indicate the flow of work within an area or process
- Document the exact time requirement for each activity within a process or area
- Display the ideal activity sequence based on takt time
- Demonstrate the time relationship between physical work (patient care, charting, dispersing medications, etc.), movement of work (transporting patients, retrieving equipment, etc.), wait times, and computer access time (retrieving a patient chart, checking doctors' orders, etc.)

The Standard Work Chart will:

- Visually display the work sequence, process layout, and work-in-process
- Visually display the staff movement for each activity, task, or process
- Visually identify quality standards, safety concerns, duplication of services, and opportunities for errors

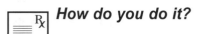 *How do you do it?*

Standard Work Combination Table

The Standard Work Combination Table is an important tool to assist management in determining work load requirements, training requirements, and potentially identifying process problems. The table clearly shows the flow of human work and all the various steps required to complete a process. Also, it will:

- Break the activity into separate elements
- Allow each element to be timed
- Allow for a good visual of the work
- Be a training tool and visual aid for the area

Standard Work Combination Table

Date	4/18	Value Stream	Dispo-to-Admit	Work (physical)	⌇
Daily Reqt.	105			Walk/Transport	⌇
Takt Time	14 minutes (avg)	Work Instruction No.	1	Computer Interaction	– –
Process Name	ED Clerk processes dispo order to wristband on patient	Page 1 of 1		Wait/Delay/Queue Time	→

Processing Times (minutes)
Wrk - Work Physical Wlk - Walk/Transport CI - Computer Interaction WT - Wait Time

# Step	Task/Activity	Wrk	Wlk	CI	WT	Processing Times chart
1	ED Clerk notes dispo in chart	0.5				
2	ED Clerk calls Bed Coord	1.0				
3	Bed Coord receives request	0.5				
4	Bed Coord checks bed status			2		
5	Bed Coord waits for bed avl				15	
6	Bed Coord cks Ns Mgr/Hskp	3.0				
7	Bed Coord confirms bed/IP	1.5				
8	Bed Coord notifies ED Clerk	1.5				
9	ED Clerk process Admit order			2.0		
10	Reg receives Admit order			0.5		
11	Reg changes pt status			2.0		
12	Reg prints new wrst/face sh	1.0				
13	Reg takes wrst/face sh to ED		4.0			
14	ED Clerk rec wrst/face sh	0.5				
15	ED Clerk places face sh	0.5				
16	ED Clerk gives wrst to Ns		4.0			
17	Ns places wrst on patient		0.5			
	Totals	10.0	8.5	6.5	15.0	

Grand Total (not including parallel waiting time, Step 5 from above) = 25.0 minutes

Standard Work Chart

The Standard Work Chart illustrates the sequence of the activities being performed. This is a very useful training tool for maintaining a standard.

It will:

- Visually convey exactly who does what and where
- Provide work instructions at the location where the activity is primarily being done to help reduce variation in the process

Standard Work Chart

Bed Request	ED Admit to Inpatient Bed Arrival
Process Name	**Value Stream**
ED	ED Staff Lounge (review only)
Department	**Posted Location**

Takt/Pitch	Upstream Process Name	Downstream Process Name
14 minutes	Dispo Written	Admit Order Written

Standard Work Sequence for: Clerk / Bed Control / Reg	Pitch Increment: N/A (Takt Time Used)

Standard Work Sequence for: Clerk / Bed Control / Reg

1. Clerk receives Dispo order
2. Clerk calls Bed Control
3. Bed Control finds bed
4. Bed Control calls Registration
5. Bed Control calls ED clerk
6. ED Clerk notes bed assignment on Dispo form
7. Registration enters admission in EMR, prints face sheet and wristband
8. Registration brings face sheet and wristband to ED clerk
9. ED clerk places face sheet in chart and gives wristband to Nurse
10. Nurse places wristband on patient
11. Patient is transported to unit

Nurse (10)

Patient Beds

Bed Control (3) (4)

(5)

(11) (9)

(2)

ED Unit Clerk (1) (6)

(8)

Registration (7)

Key Points for Standard Work in Healthcare

- Videotaping can be used to accurately document a current process. Further analysis with the Lean project team requires reviewing the video footage and documenting the various steps on the Standard Work Combination Table form.
- The Standard Work Combination Table and Standard Work Chart times can be improved upon through Kaizen Events. (See Kaizen Events)
- Both documents should be posted at the work area.
- Both documents are excellent training tools.

Case Studies and/or Photos

Bloodstream Infections

A hospital experienced an increase in systemic (bloodstream) infections. A Lean team was formed to gather additional data and problem solve. The Lean team had learned that direct observation is a powerful method for problem identification and resolution. Through observation, the increase in systemic infections was found to be due to a lack of hand washing, use of improper cleaning techniques, and difficulty removing gloves from the packaged sterile kits.

The hospital rewrote the instructions and created standard work instructions for inserting catheters and dressing changes to make them easier for staff to understand. The staff were re-trained on hand hygiene and correct cleaning methods. To eliminate the problem with the gloves, the hospital began pur-chasing a sterile glove of a higher quality. These actions dras-tically reduced the systemic infection rate. This resulted in the following outcomes:

1. Improved patient safety by drastically reducing the inci-dence of systemic infections
2. Reduction in cost ($25,000 is the average cost to treat a systemic (bloodstream) infection

Takt Time

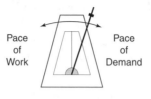

Pace of Work　　　Pace of Demand

Why use it?

Takt Time determines how fast work must proceed through the value stream to meet (customer or patient) demand.

Who does it?

The Lean project team must collect real time data or utilize historical data. (See Measurement Techniques)

How long will it take?

This should take only a few minutes to calculate. Collecting historical data may take a few hours. The time to collect real time data varies.

What does it do?

Establishing takt time for an organization will accomplish the following:

- Align work efforts to actual demand
- Focus staff awareness on what is expected
- Set a standard pace (rate) for a process (as long as other Lean tools are utilized)

How do you do it?

1. Gather appropriate data on demand.

Distribution Report				
Department Laboratory		Date January 1 - March 31		
Value Streams	January	February	March	Total
Radiology	450	575	475	1500
Floors	250	330	280	860
Pediatrics	54	48	22	124

2. Determine available work time.

Available hours of operation: Total hours available

Shifts:	1 @ 8 hours =	480 minutes
(-) Breaks:	2 @ 15 minutes per =	30 minutes
	Available working time =	450 minutes

3. Determine total daily volume required.

Lab Orders Radiology 3 months	= 1500
(/) Working days 20 per month x 3 months =	60
Average draws per day	= 25

4. Calculate takt time.

Example for Laboratory Radiology value stream:

$$\text{Takt time} = \frac{\text{Available daily work time}}{\text{Total daily volume required}} = \frac{\text{Time}}{\text{Volume}} = \frac{(T)}{(V)}$$

$$\text{Takt time} = \frac{450 \text{ minutes}}{25 \text{ blood draws}} = \textbf{18 minute takt time}$$

The 18 minute takt time is the time in which the lab has to provide the service. Takt time for this value stream must be balanced with the requirements of the other value streams to ensure people, equipment, and resources are scheduled appropriately.

Once takt time has been established, all efforts will then be required to meet the demand. This is accomplished by continuing to apply Lean tools. (See Leveling)

Note: Areas or departments that process information (i.e., supplies, labs, or radiographs) often use pitch. Takt times are used to calculate pitch, which is a more reasonable period of time to move work or provide a service throughout the value stream. (See Pitch)

Key Points for Takt Time in Healthcare

- Takt time is the rate of a service or unit of work that a facility or department must provide to meet a specific demand.
- Lean Healthcare is based on establishing accurate takt times (and pitch determinations). (See Pitch)
- Takt time (and pitch) will set the pace of work for the facility or department.
- Takt time must be calculated before standard work can be completed. (See Standard Work)
- As work volume increases and decreases, takt time must be adjusted so that staff capacity is synchronized with demand.
- Make takt time visible to the staff.

Value Stream Mapping

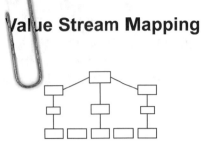

Why use it?

Value stream mapping allows a team to easily "see" the work flow and information required for a specified set of processes linked by a common theme (i.e., following a patient or work through a series of processes).

Who does it?

A cross-functional team made up of representatives of the value stream (it may also include the most downstream customer).

How long will it take?

This should take 1 to 2 days to create a current state map and a first attempt at creating a future state value stream map.

What does it do?

Value stream mapping accomplishes the following:

- Creates a common vision for everyone who is connected to the targeted value stream
- Provides a visual roadmap for the team to allocate the appropriate resources
- Provides the foundation on which to build a Lean facility

When implementing a Lean system, utilize value stream mapping in a systematic way. Do not use this tool strictly for management, get all the people involved in the exercise. Share the maps by posting them in appropriate areas.

How do you do it?

Value stream maps are of two types (or phases): the creation of the current state map and the creation of the future state map.

The current state map

Value stream mapping begins with the current state and proceeds according to the following steps:

1. Utilize icons to draw a "shell" of your current state. List the main processes, patients, customers, suppliers - internal or external. If necessary, create icons of your own that have specific meaning to the organization.

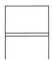 *Dedicated Process Box* - the main process or area where value-added and/or non value- added work occurs (e.g., admissions, surgery, medical records, billing, etc.)

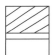 *Shared Process Box* - where multiple value streams all interrelate (e.g., labs, central supply, mail rooms, human resources, etc.)

Attribute Area - features or characteristics of the process within the process (e.g., cycle times, number of staff, mistakes (or errors), number of shifts, etc.)

 Customer or Supplier (i.e., patient, physician, vendor, etc.) - the upstream and downstream customer or supplier, with its respective attributes

Truck Shipment/Arrival - denotes the physical arrival or departure of work related to the value stream (e.g., transporting linen, supplies, ambulances, etc.)

Helicopter Shipment/Arrival - denotes the physical arrival or departure of work related to the value stream (e.g., organs, patients, etc.)

Inventory/Wait Time - the amount of time, work, people, or information that resides between two processes

Database Interaction - the time spent on computer processing

Manual Information Flow - physical conveyance of work or patients between two processes within the value stream (e.g., hand carrying work to another area, transporting patient, etc.)

Electronic Information Flow - the electronic signal that communicates information from database to process or from database to database

Mail - the arrival or sending of metered mail

Folder - a single unit of work

Folders - multiple units of work (labs, orders, charts, etc.) grouped together and moved through a common process

 Exceptions or disruptions - any major obstacle that prevents flow from occurring throughout the value stream

Go-See Scheduling - the physical viewing and collecting of information on the processes to determine work loads (e.g., charge nurse assessing staff work loads)

 Push - the movement of the patient, work, or information downstream regardless of need

 Staff - the employee assigned to the particular process

2. Go to the various areas, beginning with the most downstream process, and collect the various attributes related to the value stream. Obtain actual data. Take a stopwatch and time the process that is being evaluated. Clearly communicate to the person involved in that process what you are doing and why.

3. Determine the amount of time that work resides between each process.

4. Determine the amount of work that arrives at each process.

5. Determine what is done with the work after the process has been completed.

6. Convey all the attributes on the current state map.

7. Draw all forms of communication, electronic and/or manual.

8. Create a step graph displaying cycle times and wait times. This is typically the value-added time and non value-added times being represented.

9. Calculate total wait times and cycle times to arrive at a total lead time. Display total wait time, along with total lead time, within a box on the current state map.

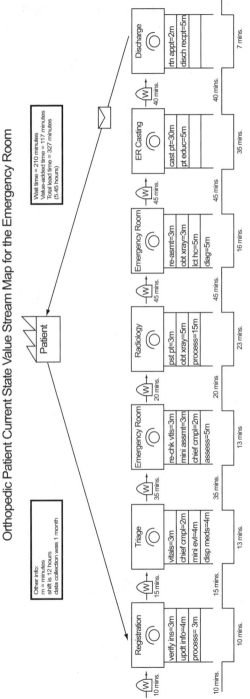

Orthopedic Patient Current State Value Stream Map for the Emergency Room

Other info:
m = minutes
shift is 12 hours
data collection was 1 month

Wait time = 210 minutes
Value-added time = 117 minutes
Total lead time = 327 minutes
(5.45 hours)

Registration
verify ins=3m
updt info=4m
process= 3m

W
15 mins.

Triage
vitals=3m
chief cmpl=2m
mini evl=4m
disp meds=4m

W
35 mins.

Emergency Room
re-chk vtls=3m
mini assmt=3m
chief cmpl=2m
assess=5m

W
20 mins.

Radiology
pst pt=3m
obt xray=5m
process=15m

W
45 mins.

Emergency Room
re-asmt=3m
obt xray=3m
lct hc=5m
diag=5m

W
45 mins.

ER Casting
cast pt=30m
pt educ=5m

W
40 mins.

Discharge
rtn appt=2m
disch recpt=5m

Patient

W
10 mins.

10 mins.

15 mins.

13 mins.

35 mins.

13 mins.

20 mins

23 mins.

45 mins

16 mins.

45 mins.

35 mins.

40 mins.

7 mins.

The following is another example of a value stream map that further separated an overall value stream into three separate ones.

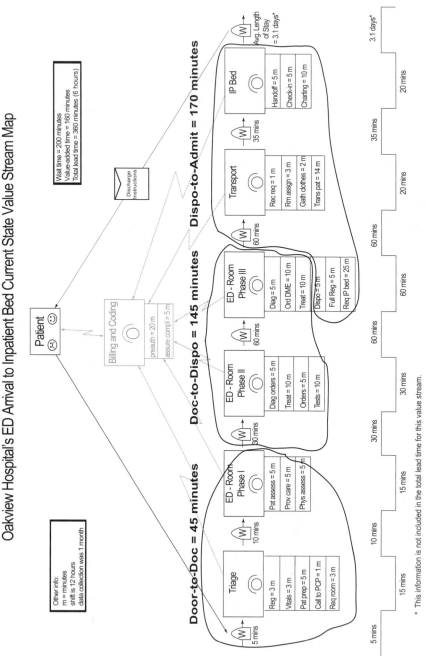

Oakview Hospital's ED Arrival to Inpatient Bed Current State Value Stream Map

THE NEW LEAN HEALTHCARE POCKET GUIDE XL

Once the map has been created, ensure that a consensus is reached with the entire team. If additional data is required, collect it now. The basis for creating a workable future state has a lot to do with the accuracy of information obtained from the current state. Do not rush this step!

Note: When creating the current state value stream map, utilize these icons as a representative sample. The team may create their own icons as appropriate.

The future state map

The future state map is the roadmap for the Lean initiatives. It is created with a team consensus, brainstorming, and simple problem solving so Lean tools are properly utilized. Additional icons that may be used are:

 Buffer Resources - temporary resources to assist work flow when there is an influx of demand (e.g., volunteers, temp workers, retirees, cross-training, overtime, etc.)

Safety Resources - temporary resources to assist work flow when there are internal issues such as turnover, illnesses, vacation, etc. (e.g., volunteers, temp workers, retirees, cross-training, overtime, etc.)

 Kaizen Event (improvement activity) - a focused group to improve a process or area within a specified time period

Cart - a device to distribute work units throughout the value stream

Kanban - work units for delivery to a process

Supermarket - an in-process location to hold work until it is required downstream

 U-shaped Work Area (cell) - the arrangement of equipment and people to accommodate efficient work flow

 Pull - the representation of work being requested from a downstream process

 FIFO - a physical location to hold work sequentially for the downstream process

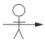 *Leveling Box* - a physical location to hold work based on volume and variety

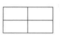 *Runner's Route* - the route the runner will use to deliver and pick-up work throughout the value stream

 Pitch Board - a physical device to hold work based on volume (e.g., a cork board or mailboxes to pick up work)

Orthopedic Patient Future State Value Stream Map for the Emergency Room

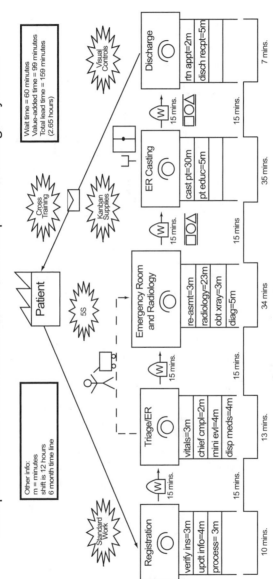

Other info:
m = minutes
shift is 12 hours
6 month time line

Wait time = 60 minutes
Value-added time = 99 minutes
Total lead time = 159 minutes
(2.65 hours)

Standard Work

Registration
verify ins=3m
updt info=4m
process= 3m
10 mins.

15 mins.

Triage/ER
vitals=3m
chief cmpl=2m
mini evl=4m
disp meds=4m
13 mins.

15 mins.

5S

Emergency Room and Radiology
re-asmt=3m
radiology=23m
obt xray=3m
diag=5m
34 mins

15 mins.

Cross Training

Kanban Supplies

Patient

ER Casting
cast pt=30m
pt educ=5m
35 mins.

15 mins.

Visual Controls

Discharge
rtn appt=2m
disch recpt=5m
7 mins.

15 mins.

The following illustration is the Dispo-to-Admit future state value stream portion as shown on page 180.

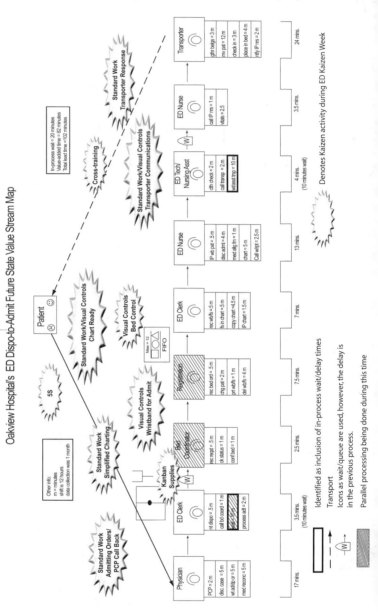

Remember, the overall goal of creating a visual aid via a value stream map is to clearly identify waste. It also enables you to obtain an accurate portrayal of current work conditions. Many times there will be some basic issues arising once the current state value stream map has been created. There may be times, for a variety of reasons, that the current state mapping needs to be postponed due to an issue or problem identified. If that is the case, address the issue or problem using a problem solving methodology. (See Problem Solving)

Key Points for Value Stream Mapping in Healthcare

- Value stream mapping is a valuable part of a systematic approach to implementing Lean.
- It is a great visual aid for identifying waste.
- You can create great maps, but the follow-through is most important. Use other Lean tools in this pocket guide to continue to implement your future state.
- Always draw the customer first and think of improvements from that perspective.
- Future state maps will have many iterations.
- Ensure key people are involved in creating the maps.

Case Studies and/or Photos

Pathology

In one hospital, physicians often would not receive anatomical pathologists' reports for four to five days. Multiple attempts had been made prior to Lean to improve this turnaround time, but they were all unsuccessful. Staff had attended a Lean conference and decided to use the value stream mapping tool to identify waste in the process. The team set a goal of a two day turnaround time. They observed the current process from receipt of the specimen to delivery of the pathology report.

A value stream map was developed and four problems were clearly identified on the current state map:

1. Paperwork did not flow with the specimen. This forced the transcriptionist to spend three to four hours per day manually matching paperwork to specimens. Existing software was changed, enabling paperwork to print in the same order as the specimen flow.
2. Scheduled work time of different areas of the lab also caused interruptions in the flow of specimens. For example, staff in the grossing area worked from 7:00 am to 6:00 pm. Specimens arriving after 6:00 pm were not touched until the following day. Histology embedding began at 5:00 am; therefore, the pathologists did not receive slides until 10:00 am. The grossing area lengthened its day to 10:00 pm to address specimens received after 6:00 pm and histology embedding began at 3:00 am in order to get slides to the pathologists by 7:30 am.
3. Transcriptionists were moved to a quieter area to decrease interruptions. This decreased report turnaround time from four or five hours to one hour.
4. Because many work processes were not standardized, labeling errors sometimes occurred that led to delays in the flow of specimens. The process was properly documented. This led to a reduction of errors from approximately three per month to one in the first 2-1/2 months of the process improvement.

The team created a future state map and the following Lean tools were used: (1) continuous flow, (2) work load balancing, (3) physical layout, and (4) standard work. This resulted in the following outcomes:

1. Reduced report turnaround time from four to five days to two days
2. Improved referring physician satisfaction by the reduction of lead time of report distribution
3. Improved safety by reducing labeling errors

Visual Controls

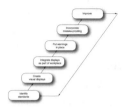

Why use it?

This will establish a visual communication system. This ensures adherence to standards so work is completed on schedule without errors.

Who does it?

The Lean project team will continually implement visual controls as part of any continuous improvement activity.

How long will it take?

This is to be reviewed continually and will never be completed. Visual controls will also be updated to reflect continuous improvement activities.

What does it do?

Visual controls in an area will accomplish the following:

- Reduce confusion
- Encourage standardization of a process
- Establish the need of visual aides (displays) to encourage staff involvement
- Improve productivity
- Reduce internal errors
- Reduce stress

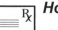 ### *How do you do it?*

The following steps can be used to create a visual language throughout the facility:

1. Form and train the visual controls team.
2. Create an implementation plan.
3. Begin implementation.
4. Ensure 5S system implementation.
5. Standardize visual measurements.
6. Standardize visual displays.
7. Standardize visual controls.

1. Form and train the visual controls team.

This may be a subset of the Lean project team. Creating this part of the Lean project can be fun to do, but it will require additional time. Many Lean project teams do not give this the appropriate time. It will be the team's responsibility to:

- Create the locations where visual displays and standards will be posted
- Establish visual measurements (VM) (i.e., bar charts, pie charts, goals, outcomes, etc.), visual displays (VD) (i.e., banners, placards, signs, etc.) and visual controls (VC) (i.e., alarms, lights, color-codes, etc.)
- Create standards for all visuals (location, updates, themes, etc.)

2. Create an implementation plan.

The core team must designate target areas with a timeline for training and implementation. Each target area may require a champion. (See Reporting and Communications)

The following Visual Control Worksheet can be utilized for the planning stage.

Visual Control Worksheet

Team Champion _____   Date _____

Department/Work Area _____

Evaluation Date	5S Completion Date	VM Completion Date	VD Completion Date	VC Completion Date

3. Begin implementation.

Once a plan has been determined for using visuals to improve an area or process, immediately deploy it. The displays or controls will be improved upon by input from staff.

4. Ensure 5S system implementation.

Work with current 5S teams to assist them with the 4th and 5th S.

5. Standardize visual measurements.

The Lean project should have identified appropriate measurements or other performance measurements critical to the facility. (See Goals and Outcomes)

Visual measurements must have the following attributes:

- Directly relate to strategy
- Be non-financial
- Be location-specific
- Be easy to collect and post
- Provide for fast feedback
- Foster improvement initiatives

The following illustration is a visual measurement of a Patient Satisfaction Survey.

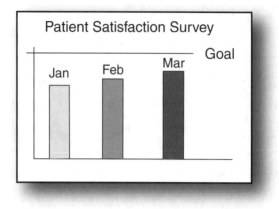

6. Standardize visual displays.

Visual displays communicate important information about the facility in terms of goals, outcomes, safety, environment, or other related activities. Signboards are often used as a visual display. Bulletin boards are often used to display this type of information.

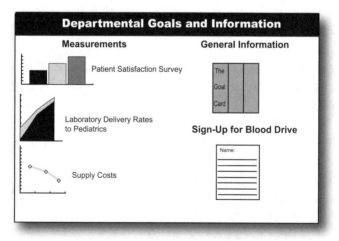

7. Standardize visual controls.

The standard created is to integrate visual measurements, visual displays, and visual controls to ensure process control. This would include task lists, checklists, and computer programs to ensure that what has been created in the visual control system is sustained (i.e., mistake proofing). (See Error Proofing)

Mistake proofing or error proofing is the designing of a process to significantly reduce or eliminate errors that cause defects.

For example: medications are being administered to a patient on the floor. To eliminate errors, the 7 Rights and Triple Check must be followed. The 7 Rights are:

1. Right patient
2. Right medications
3. Right dose
4. Right route
5. Right time
6. Right technique
7. Right documentation

Many times an 8th Right will include patient education.

The Triple Check is:

1. Check medication as you take it off the shelf
2. Check medication as you prepare it
3. Check medication as you replace it on the shelf

A visual display can be the listing of the 7 Rights and Triple Check on the medication cart or on the cabinet where the medications are stored. A visual control can be a fingerprint or your ID card scanned on a reader prior to accessing the medications.

The following illustration displays the progression for using and implementing visual controls.

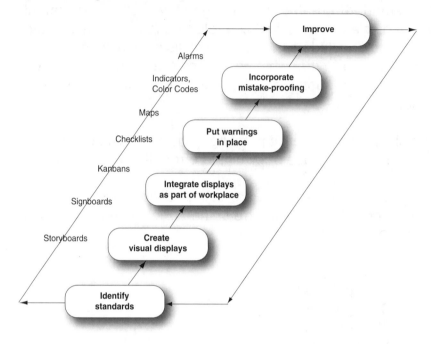

The following chart lists various types of visual displays and controls that can be used.

General Purpose	
Storyboards	Share information about projects or improvements Educate and motivate
Signboards	Share vital information at point-of-use
Maps	Share actual processes, standard operating procedures, directions, etc.
Kanbans	Control the withdrawal of work (or supplies) in and out of supermarkets, work areas, etc. Can be used to regulate work in FIFO lanes
Checklists	Provide an operational tool that facilitates adherence to standards, procedures, etc.
Indicators, Color Codes	Show correct location, item types, amount, or direction of work flow
Alarms	Provide a strong, unavoidable sign or signal when action needs to be taken (email alert, text message, pager code, etc.)

Key Points for Visual Controls in Healthcare

- One picture is worth a thousand words. This is what visual control is about. If a picture, diagram, or digital photo is exactly where you need it and when you need it, it will ensure a standard is met. Therefore, it is well worth the time and effort.
- Visual displays and controls should be part of all Lean tool applications.
- Visuals should begin with the first Lean project team meeting by posting the Team Charter and Meeting Information Form. (See Reporting and Communications)
- Visual controls are Just-In-Time information. (See Just-In-Time)
- Ensure visual controls are updated regularly and are part of the facility audit process.

Case Studies and/or Photos

Adult Immunizations

A hospital's staff was not meeting its goal to screen and pro-vide the pneumovax and influenza vaccines to 100% of eligible patients. Prior to implementing Lean, screening and adminis-tration of the vaccines occurred on the day of discharge. Patients' discharges were often delayed by 15 minutes on average because they had to wait for the medications to be delivered. Sometimes, patients refused to wait and left without their immunizations. The original order form had the standing order at the bottom of the page, where it was often overlooked. The staff members reviewed the standing order form using the Lean concept of visual controls. They decided to place the order at the top of the page with clear instructions. As a result of this visual control, the immunizations are now stored nearer the dispensing point and may be accessed and administered immediately. These improvements helped this hospital's staff improve and maintain outstanding pneumovax and influenza vaccination rates. This resulted in the following outcomes:

1. Reduced the wait time for immunizations to less than 3 minutes
2. Reduced non value-added steps in the process from 15 to 8
3. Improved immunization rates from 31% to 100% compli-ant

Bed Control

The Bed Control Manager wanted a better way to indicate to physicians that the hospital was nearing capacity. Although an email was sent each morning indicating the capacity status, not all physicians monitored their emails closely. A small team, including the Physician Relations Manager, installed a visual "stop light" at two key physician locations: the physician lounge and the hospital entrance nearest the physician parking lot. Colored circles were placed on the stoplight as follows: Green, less than 75% of beds filled; Orange, 76 - 85% of beds filled; and Red, 86% or more of beds filled.

ED

When ED patients were ready to be transferred to their inpatient units, or discharged, the nurses sometimes had difficulty locating charts, even though they were supposedly completed. It turned out that sometimes physicians or residents would take the charts to add a comment, or check results. A small group of ED team members created a "STOP - DO NOT REMOVE" sign to be placed on the chart when the ED documentation was completed. They asked for cooperation from the residents and physicians to add any comments or check results right at the patient's bedside, leaving the chart always near the patient for the nurse to find when needed.

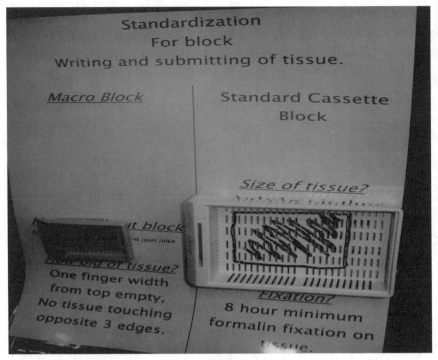

Biopsy tissues samples submitted to the laboratory are placed in a plastic cassette, processed, and then further embedded in wax for cutting to be added on a slide for diagnostic interpretation. Standard work, along with visual aids, was developed due to multiple variations in specimen processing that included: tissue size and correct placement in the cassette for further processing.

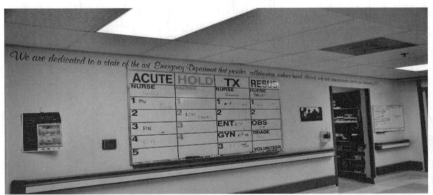

Located near the unit clerk's desk, this large patient peg board denotes the patient status in the ED. Now, everyone knows where all patients are in the process.

THE NEW LEAN HEALTHCARE POCKET GUIDE XL

Waste

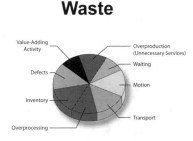

 Why use it?

It is used to identify, analyze, and eliminate all non value-added activities by utilizing Lean tools and practices. Waste is anything that adds cost or time without adding value.

Who does it?

The elimination of waste and variation is the foundation of Lean. All staff are to identify and work to eliminate waste.

How long will it take?

The process is never-ending. (See Predictable Output)

 What does it do?

Anything that adds cost or time without adding value is waste. Eliminating waste will accomplish the following:

- Improve patient care and safety
- Reduce cost to the facility
- Reduce wait time between processes
- Improve productivity
- Improve quality
- Make the facility more competitive
- Encourage teamwork and staff involvement

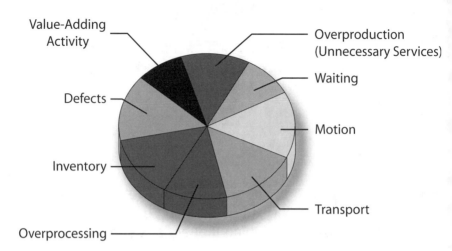

Value-Adding Activity

Overproduction (Unnecessary Services)

Waiting

Defects

Motion

Inventory

Transport

Overprocessing

How do you do it?

The process of waste elimination can be applied to any process or value stream. The following areas of waste will be explained with reference to the various Lean tools and practices. These tools can be used in the identification and elimination of waste.

1. The Waste of Overproduction (Unnecessary Services)

This waste is producing work or providing a service prior to it being required or requested. That is the greatest of all the wastes. If you overproduce some type of work or service, it encompasses many of the other wastes. For example, dietary may send extra meal trays when a patient has been discharged or moved to another floor or unit. This would include waste in: excessive processing, transport, motion, overproduction, etc.

Examples of overproduction wastes are:

- Treatment (meds, dressing changes, etc.) given early to suit staff schedule
- Testing ahead of time to suit lab schedule
- Treatments done not on schedule but instead at times to accommodate hospital staff/equipment capacity
- Making extra copies of charts, reports, labs, etc.
- Printing, emailing, sending, or faxing the same document multiple times
- Entering repetitive information on documents or forms

To eliminate this type of waste, you will use the following Lean tools:

- Takt Time
- Measurement Techniques
- Pitch
- Standard Work
- Leveling
- Predictable Output
- Continuous Flow
- Pull Systems
- Others as appropriate

2. The Waste of Waiting

Waiting for anything, be it people, equipment, signatures, supplies, or information, is waste. This waste of waiting is "low hanging fruit." It is easy to identify and "ripe for the taking." We often do not think of paper sitting in an "In-basket" as waste. However, when looking for an item, how many times do we search through the In-basket to find it? This is identified as a time waster. How many times do you actually touch something before you complete the task? The "finish, file, or throw it away" system can help with eliminating this waste.

Examples of waiting wastes are:

- Delays for bed assignments
- Waiting for admissions to ER
- Excessive signatures or approvals
- Delays for lab test results
- Delays in receiving information or patients
- Cross-departmental resource commitments
- Patient back-up due to equipment not working properly or not available

To eliminate this type of waste, you will use the following Lean tools:

- Value Stream Mapping
- 5S
- Measurement Techniques
- Reporting and Communications
- Pitch
- Work Load Balancing
- Runner
- Kaizen Events
- Paper File System
- Others as appropriate

3. The Waste of Motion (excess)

Any excess movement of people, equipment, paper information, or electronic exchanges (e-mails, etc.) that does not add value is waste. This waste can be created by poor physical layout or design, which can be responsible for more walking, reaching, or bending than necessary.

Examples of motion wastes are:

- Searching for patients
- Searching for charts and/or doctor's orders
- Searching for medications and/or equipment
- Hand-carrying paperwork to another process
- Searching for poorly located supplies

To eliminate this type of waste, you will use the following Lean tools:

- Standard Work
- 5S
- Physical Layout
- Document Tagging
- Paper File System
- Kanbans for Supplies
- Pull Systems
- Others as appropriate

4. The Waste of Transport (or excess Conveyance)

Transport is an important and ubiquitous element. It affects the delivery of any work within a facility. It is the excess movement of work that does not add value.

Examples of transport wastes are:

- Transporting the surgical patient from an outpatient area to preop prior to surgery
- Placing a gurney in the hall and constantly having to move it
- Moving samples, specimens, or equipment early or late to the wrong location

To eliminate this type of waste, you will use the following Lean tools:

- Standard Work
- 5S
- Physical Layout
- Document Tagging
- Runners
- Paper File System
- Continuous Flow
- Kaizen Events
- Others as appropriate

5. The Waste of Overprocessing

Putting more work or effort into things that a patient, physician, healthcare provider, etc. does not want or ask for is waste. Overprocessing does not add value and the customer will not want to pay for it.

Examples of overprocessing wastes are:

- Ordering more diagnostic tests than the diagnosis warrants (i.e., ordering a Chem 24 when a Chem 6 will suffice or replacing a heparin lock before policy dictates it to be changed)
- Requesting and processing information that will never be used
- Entering repetitive information

To eliminate this type of waste, you will use the following Lean tools:

- Value Stream Mapping
- Standard Work
- Document Tagging
- Reporting and Communications
- Work Load Balancing
- Measurement Techniques
- Kaizen Events
- Visual Controls
- Others as appropriate

6. The Waste of Inventory

Excess stock, work piles, and supplies are waste. They all take up space. Note: time is considered excess inventory if it is not used efficiently.

Examples of inventory wastes are:

- Duplicate medications and supplies in excess of normal usage
- Extra or outdated manuals, newsletters, or magazines
- Excessive office supplies
- Obsolete charts, files, and equipment
- Patients in waiting rooms
- Insufficient cross-training of staff

To eliminate this type of waste, you will use the following Lean tools:

- 5S
- Value Stream Mapping
- Standard Work
- Visual Controls
- Pull Systems
- Kanbans for Supplies
- Others as appropriate

7. The Waste of Defects

This category of waste refers to all processing required to correct a defect or mistake. Defects (either internal or external) result in additional processes (and possible services) that will add no value to the product or service. The idea is that it takes a shorter time to do it correctly the first time than it does to do it over to correct the problem.

Examples of defect wastes are:

- Retesting (i.e., performing a second 24-hour urine test because a staff member obtained the first specimen incorrectly)
- Medication errors
- Wrong patient information
- Wrong procedure
- Missing information

To eliminate this type of waste, you will use the following Lean tools:

- Error Proofing
- 5S
- Standard Work
- Predictable Output
- Visual Controls
- Paper File System
- Interruptions and Random Arrivals
- Others as appropriate

8. The Waste of Unused Creativity

You will also find an eighth waste - unused creativity. This waste does not utilize the available talents and skills of staff to their fullest.

Examples of unused creativity are:

- No defined performance management system
- Little or no cross-training

To eliminate this type of waste, you will use the following Lean tools:

- Develop a performance management system
- Create training and development plans for each employee

This was a quick review of the wastes, with examples for consideration. Consider the following questions:

1. "How can I start to communicate about these wastes throughout the department or facility?" (What are the quick and obvious wastes that can be easily addressed?)
2. "What are some low-hanging fruit?"
3. "What can be done immediately to improve patient, provider, and staff satisfaction?"

These types of question should stimulate similar questions and allow for open communications regarding waste.

Key Points for Waste in Healthcare

- Waste is anything that does not add value to the patient, healthcare provider, or staff.
- Waste must be viewed with "fresh" eyes. Invite other departments to meetings to help brainstorm. This may assist in waste identification and elimination.
- Waste should be looked at from both the macro (facility or value stream) level and the micro (task/activity) level.
- The root of all waste is variation from a process standard.
- Identification and elimination of waste must be a daily activity throughout the facility by all personnel. And when this occurs, then, and only then, will a continuous improvement culture emerge.

Work Load Balancing

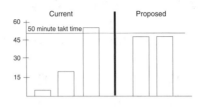

 ## Why use it?

This determines how to distribute work units (activities) across the value stream to meet takt time or pitch.

Note: this may not apply to all areas of the facility due to certifications, licensing, training, etc.

For example, nurses are staffed according to the number of patients and level of care needed for a shift. This is adjusted as circumstances change. As more critical patients arrive, the work load has to be adjusted. This is a form of Work Load Balancing. This section will demonstrate a visual method to do this.

Who does it?

The Lean project team with representation from the area or process being improved.

How long will it take?

It will take approximately 4 - 8 hours to analyze current work duties and brainstorm for improvements. 1 – 2 weeks to plan, create standards, and train.

What does it do?

Work load balancing will accomplish the following:

- Evenly distribute work units
- Obtain accurate cycle times for each process
- Define the order that process steps are completed
- Define the number of staff required for a given demand
- Assist in creating the future state map
- Improve productivity

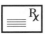 ## How do you do it?

Work load balancing begins with an analysis of your current state. The best tool to perform this is the Employee Balance Chart.

Employee Balance Chart

The Employee Balance Chart is a visual representation of process activities in the form of a bar chart. It represents work duties and activities. It can be used to determine how to balance the work within the value stream. There are seven steps to creating the Employee Balance Chart. The seven steps are:

1. Visually display the list of processes from the current state value stream map.
2. Obtain individual cycle times for the various process activities.
3. Add the individual cycle times to obtain total cycle time.
4. Create the Employee Balance Chart of the current state.
5. Determine the ideal number of staff.
6. Create the Employee Balance Chart of the future state.
7. Re-allocate work duties, train, and document.

1. Visually display the list of processes from the current state value stream map.

Be very clear about identifying the process, beginning and end. Be explicit to the process's parameters. The team should have a good handle of the processes from creating the value stream map. (See Value Stream Mapping)

2. Obtain individual cycle times for the various process activities.

These cycle times should be derived from the current state value stream map. Re-visit these times to ensure their accuracy. Team members may want to take a stopwatch and time the various tasks within the process.

For example, these are process cycle times for a medical clinic's new patient exam value stream:

Registration	15 minutes
Medical Assistant Prep	4 minutes
Pre-post provider visit (RN)	5 minutes
Evaluation/Diagnosis (physician or PA)	6 minutes

3. Add the individual cycle times to obtain the total cycle time. (See Cycle Time)

From the above example, the total cycle time would be the individual cycle times of 15, 4, 5, and 6 minutes. This is a total cycle time of 30 minutes.

4. Create the Employee Balance Chart of the current state.

Make a bar chart identifying each process and staff, along with the various individual cycle times. It is recommended that you visually display the chart on a easel with a flip chart so the team can review it as a group and comment. Use Post-it Notes to represent the tasks associated with the processes. Make the Post-it Notes proportional to the time element for each individual task. Draw a horizontal line to represent takt time. (See Takt Time)

For this example, the medical clinic has established the takt time to be 12 minutes. Over the course of 3 months, they averaged 35 new patient visits per day. The available working time per day was 420 minutes; therefore, the takt time was 12 minutes per exam (420 minutes divided by 35 exams).

Notice that each task is further broken down into segments representing activities to completing that task.

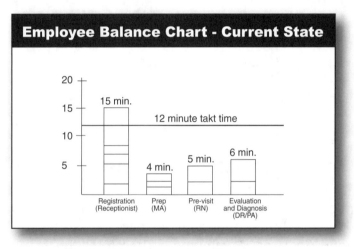

5. Determine the ideal number of staff.

To determine the ideal number of staff needed to meet the requirements of the value stream: divide the total process cycle time by the takt time. (See Cycle Time)

To continue with this example, the total process cycle time is 30 minutes, which is divided by the 12 minute takt time. This equates to 2.5 staff. Remember, this is only for this value stream. The staff most likely will have other value streams in which they must work in throughout the day.

6. Create the Employee Balance Chart of the future state.

Work with the team and move the Post-it Notes around to balance the various work duties. Work to have each staff member balanced to takt time, while maintaining the flow of work.

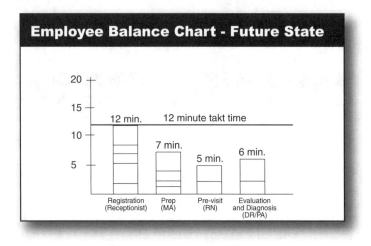

From our previous new patient exam value stream, it was visually conveyed that the receptionist could not keep up with the demand (takt) of 12 minutes. Therefore, the medical clinic team decided that the MA could assist the process by phoning for the insurance information, which was the 3 minute element of the receptionists' process time. These three minutes allowed the value stream to be better balanced.

7. Re-allocate work duties, train, and document.

Once a consensus has been obtained on balancing the duties, create standard work.

In summary work load balancing will:

- Evenly distribute work duties among the staff
- Define the order work duties are performed
- Define the number of staff required
- Assist in the physical layout design

Key Points for Work Load Balancing in Healthcare

- Ensure accurate cycle times are established.
- Do not eliminate people, but utilize them in other value stream areas.
- Utilize visual controls when training.
- Establish the best method for a process.

Case Studies and/or Photos

Laboratory

A laboratory pursued Lean because it was performing in the lower quartile of productivity and cost per test. The physicians and nursing staff were also dissatisfied with the turnaround time of test results.

Two major changes were implemented to reach the goal of reporting 95% of test results within 30 minutes of when the specimen was drawn. First was the change to consolidate two separate rooms with six separate workstations into one automated work cell designed to enable one person to operate six separate work stations. The second change was the implementation of a one-piece flow phlebotomy process to increase the number of specimens a phlebotomist could handle per hour. The results were:

1. Reduced turnaround time of lab results by 50%
2. Improved productivity by more than 40%
3. Reduced costs by 31%
4. Saved more than 440 square feet of space

Glossary of Lean Healthcare Terms

5S - A process to ensure work areas are systematically kept clean and organized, ensuring employee safety, and providing the foundation on which to build a Lean culture.

Active state - The horizontal position of a file folder indicating work needs to be completed.

Activity - The single or multiple act of taking a course of action.

Assessment - A structured form upon which to analyze a department or area relative to a particular topic.

Benchmarking - A structured approach to identify, visit, and adapt world-class practices to an organization.

Brainstorming - The process of capturing people's ideas and organizing those thoughts around common themes.

Catchball - The back and forth communication between levels within an organization to ensure team alignment.

Cause and effect diagram - The visual representation to clearly display the various factors affecting a process.

Champion - The person that has authority to commit resources for the facility. Also referred to as Team Champion.

Check sheet - The visual representation of the times an activity, event, or process occurred over a time period.

Continuous flow - A process's ability to replenish a single work unit or service that has been requested or "pulled" from a downstream process. It is synonymous with Just-In-Time (JIT), which ensures both internal and external customers receive the work unit or service when it is needed, in the exact amounts.

Control chart - The visual representation of tracking progress over time. Similar to line graphs.

Control point - A physical element of work within a process that has clearly set limits. For example, the minimum and maximum levels for the office supplies would be control points.

Cross training - The process to convey work competencies to other employees to better utilize resources.

Cycle time - The time elapsed from the beginning of a work process request until it is completed.

Customer - The patient, person, and/or process that requires a service and is paying for it.

Customer demand - The quantity of product or service required by the customer. Also referred to as takt time.

Data - Factual information used as a basis for further analysis.

Delay time - The time element between two processes. Also referred to as wait or queue time.

Document tagging - The physical attachment of a form to a process work unit to document dates and times.

Downstream - The patient, provider, and/or process that a request or service to being provided to.

Elapsed time - The delay time plus the cycle time.

First-In First-Out (FIFO) - The work controlled method to ensure the oldest work upstream (first-in) is the first to be processed downstream (first-out). This could be a raised flag or an e-mail alert.

Fishbone diagram - *See Cause and effect diagram*

Flow - The movement of material or information.

Frequency chart - The visual representation of the number of times an activity, event, or process occurred for a specified time period.

Goal - The end result to which effort is directed.

Goal Card - The document displaying the strategic mission of the organization, along with departmental, team, and/or individual goals.

Group cycle time - The rate of completing a group task or objective. It is the total individual cycle times added together for a project.

Heijunka (same as Leveling) - The balancing of work amongst the workers during a period of time, both by volume and variety.

Heijunka box - A physical device to hold the work units arranged by value streams. Similar to a group of mail boxes.

Histogram - The visual representation that displays the spread and shape of the data distribution.

Individual cycle time - The rate of completion of an individual task or single operation of work.

In-process supermarket - The control of work units in and out of an area residing between two processes to improve work flow.

Interruption - The stopping of a process without notice.

Just-In-Time (JIT) - Synonymous with continuous flow. It is the provision that the process or customer is supplied with the exact product or service, with the right amount, at the right time.

Kaizen - "Kai" means to "take apart" and "zen" means to "make good." Kaizen is synonymous with continuous improvement.

Kaizen Event - A focused group of individuals dedicated to applying Lean tools to a specific area within a certain time period.

Kanban - A card or visual indicator that serves as a means of communicating to an upstream process precisely what is required at the specified time.

Lean healthcare - The application of the Toyota Production System tools and concepts to the healthcare industry.

Leveling - See Heijunka.

Leveling or Heijunka Box - The physical device that contains the service or work request based on value stream requirements.

Metric - A specific number (data) that is utilized to measure before and after improvement initiatives.

Meeting Information Form - The document to effectively manage meetings, detail agendas, and list action items.

Multi-disciplinary team - The staff, who are working on a continuous improvement project, that have different skills.

Non value-added - The part of the process that the customer will not pay for. Also referred to as waste.

Office layout - A self-contained, well-occupied space that improves the flow of work and data transactions. This would include software requirements.

Outcome - The result of identifying and eliminating waste.

Owner - The staff member who is responsible for assuring the process is standardized to best practice.

Paper file system - The methodology of grouping and organizing all paperwork and staff skills to eliminate waste.

Pareto chart - The visual representation in a bar chart format listing issues in descending order of importance.

Passive state - The vertical position of a file folder indicating work has been completed.

Pitch - The adjusted takt time to move work units throughout the value stream.

Predictable output - The assurance that a work unit or service will be exactly what is expected.

Problem solving - A team working together, following a structured process, to remedy a situation that caused a deviation from a norm.

Process - The sequence of tasks (or activities) to deliver a product or service.

Process folder - The specific information and detailed flow for a particular process.

Process mapping - The visual representation of a sequence of operations (tasks) consisting of people, work duties, and transactions that occur for the design and delivery of a product or service.

Process master document - The listing of all processes within a department or value stream.

Process owner - *See Owner.*

Project champion - *See Champion*

Pull - A system in which nothing is produced by the upstream (supplier process) until the downstream (customer process) signals the need for it. This enables work to flow without detailed schedules.

Push - The work that is pushed along regardless of need or request.

Queue times - The amount of time a work unit or service request must wait before it is released.

Random arrival - The interruption of a process by another process or person.

Red tag - A label used in the 5S process to identify items that are not needed or are placed in the wrong area.

Resistance - The opposition of an idea or concept.

Root cause - The origin or source of the problem.

Runner - A designated staff member whose function is to maintain value stream pitch integrity.

Scatter and concentration plots - The visual representation of data to study the possible relationship between one variable and another.

Set-In-Order - The second activity in the 5S system. This will ensure items are properly stored and placed in the correct location.

Shine - The third activity in the 5S system. This involves cleaning everything thoroughly and ensuring cleaning is part of the audit process.

Six Sigma - The measure of variation that achieves 3.4 defects per million opportunities, or 99.99966 percent acceptable.

Sort - The first activity in the 5S system. This is the weeding out of items within the target area that have not been used for a period of time or are not expected to be used.

Simplified folder system - A process to ensure work is organized and processed correctly, thus becoming a basis for improvement activities.

Standardize - The fourth activity in the 5S system. This involves the creation of documents/rules to ensure the first 3 S's will be done regularly (and made visible).

Standard work - This is a process to gather the relevant information to document the best practice of producing a work unit or providing a service. It should be the basis for all continuous improvement activities.

Standard Work Combination Table - The visual representation displaying the flow of human work and all the various steps required to complete a process.

Standard Work Chart - The visual representation displaying the sequence, process layout, and work units for a process.

Status Report - The document to detail the team's progress to date, as well as issues and plans to keep on track.

Storyboard - A graphically rich, visual representation of a Lean or problem solving project that displays critical information. Storyboards can be 8.5" x 11" or can be poster size.

Supermarket - The system to store a certain level of in-process work or service capacity to be pulled by the downstream customer when there is a difference in the cycle times of the process(es).

Supplier - The provider of a service or work unit to a down-stream process.

Sustain - The fifth activity in the 5S system. This involves the process of monitoring and ensuring adherence to the first 4 S's. Many times this will be a regular audit.

System folder - The "keeper" of all pertinent information about the processes within a department or value stream.

Takt time - The pace of customer demand. Takt time determines how fast a process must run to meet customer demand.

Task - A single event within a process.

Team Charter - A document detailing the team's mission and proposed outcomes to ensure strategic alignment.

Total cycle time - The rate of completion of a process or group of tasks that have a common element. It is calculated by adding up the individual cycle times for that process or value stream.

Upstream process - The provider of a service or work unit required downstream from a customer.

Value-Added Time Reporting Log - The document to track the process cycle times.

Value-added time - The time element that the customer is willing to pay for. This time should be void of waste.

Value stream - A sequence of processes that are connected by a common customer, product, or service request.

Value stream mapping - The visual representation of the processes (work units and information required) to meet a customer demand.

Visual control - The visual indicators used to ensure a process produces what is expected, and if not, what must happen.

Visual metric - The display of measurements.

Visual office - The ability to convey all relevant information about a product or service by the means of signs, posters, and/or anything that appears to the eye.

Waste - Anything that adds cost or time without adding value. The seven most common wastes are: 1) Overproducing, 2) Waiting, 3) Transport, 4) Overprocessing, 5) Inventory, 6) Motion, and 7) Defects. Many times you will see an eighth waste added, 8) Unused Creativity.

Work load balancing - The distribution of work units across the value stream to meet takt time or pitch.

Work unit - A specific, measurable amount of work that can be segmented and treated as a whole. For example, lab reports, physician orders, charts, insurance claims, etc.

Index

5 Whys 127
5S 1, 212
5S Area Audit 10
5S Cleaning Plan 7
5S Training Matrix 10

A
Active state 212
Active state folder 99
Adult Immunizations 194
Assessment 212

B
Bed Control 195
Bedside Pumps 137
Benchmarking 212
Black Belt 162
Bloodstream Infections 171
Brainstorming 133, 212

C
Catchball 47, 212
Cause and effect diagram 130, 212
Champion 73-74, 147-148, 152, 156, 188, 212, 217
Check Sheets 130, 166, 212
Continuous flow 18-19, 21, 23-25, 69, 85, 107, 112, 141, 186, 199, 201, 212, 214
Control chart 213
Couriers 90
Criteria Checklist for Set-In-Order 5
Critical 99
Cross training 213
CT 30
Customer demand 213
Cycle Time 26, 213

D

Data 213
Data Capture Form 92-93
Defect 38, 161, 203
Delay time 213
Distribution Report 94
Document Tagging 31, 213
Document Tagging Worksheet 32
Downstream 213

E

ED 83, 144, 195
Elapsed time 213
Emergency Department 56
Employee Balance Chart 207-208, 210

F

Facilities 118
Failure Prevention Analysis Worksheet 38
First-In First-Out (FIFO) 18, 21-25, 84, 112, 141-142, 145, 182, 213
Fishbone Diagrams 130, 213
Five Minute 5S Checklist 8
Flow 214
Flowcharts 128
Frequency chart 214

G

Goal Card 50-51, 214
Goals 45, 53

H

Heijunka 85, 214
Histogram 132, 214
Hyperbaric Medicine 63

I

Individual cycle time 27, 214
In-Process Supermarkets 18-20, 22-23, 112, 141-142
Interruption Log 66-67
Inventory waste 81
Is/Is Not 125

J

Just-In-Time (JIT) 68-70, 82, 212, 214

K

Kaizen 71, 215
Kaizen Event 29, 71-75, 171, 200-202, 215
Kaizen Milestone Worksheet 73-74
Kanban 19, 102, 215
Kanban card 80

L

Lab 44, 90
Laboratory 211
Level 1 - Indicators 41
Level 2 - Signals 41
Level 3 - Physical or Electronic Controls 41
Leveling 85, 87
Leveling Sequence Table 87, 91

M

Measurement Techniques 92-95, 113, 172, 199-200, 202
Meeting Information Form 150, 215
Metric 215
Mistake-Proofing 36, 191
Motion waste 88, 112, 114
Multi-disciplinary team 215

N

Non value-added 215
Non-critical 99
Nosocomial Infections 42

U

Unused creativity 204, 220
Upstream process 219

V

Value Stream Mapping 175, 219
Value-added time 219
Value-Added Time Reporting Log 105, 219
Visual aids 25, 116, 122, 142, 157
Visual control 38, 40, 41, 142-143, 188, 191, 193-194, 219
Visual displays 188, 190-191, 193
Visual measurements 188-189, 191
Visual metric 220

W

Waiting 199
Waiting waste 24
Waste 197, 220
Work Load Balancing 206, 220
Work unit 220

Z

Zero defects 36, 42, 161